WHEEL

A RECOVERY FROM CHRONIC PAIN AND
DISCOVERY OF NEW ENERGY

Sylvia Hawthorn-Deppen

BALBOA.
PRESS
A DIVISION OF HAY HOUSE

Balboa Press books may be ordered through booksellers or by contacting:

Balboa Press
A Division of Hay House
1663 Liberty Drive
Bloomington, IN 47403
www.balboapress.com
1-(877) 407-4847

Because of the dynamic nature of the Internet, any web addresses or links contained in this book may have changed since publication and may no longer be valid. The views expressed in this work are solely those of the author and do not necessarily reflect the views of the publisher, and the publisher hereby disclaims any responsibility for them.

The author of this book does not dispense medical advice or prescribe the use of any technique as a form of treatment for physical, emotional, or medical problems without the advice of a physician, either directly or indirectly. The intent of the author is only to offer information of a general nature to help you in your quest for emotional and spiritual well-being. In the event you use any of the information in this book for yourself, which is your constitutional right, the author and the publisher assume no responsibility for your actions.

Any people depicted in stock imagery provided by Thinkstock are models, and such images are being used for illustrative purposes only.
Certain stock imagery © Thinkstock.

ISBN: 978-1-4525-5565-2 (sc)
ISBN: 978-1-4525-5566-9 (hc)
ISBN: 978-1-4525-5564-5 (e)

Library of Congress Control Number: 2012913023

Printed in the United States of America

Balboa Press rev. date: 10/05/2012

Contents

Dedication xi

Foreword...xiii

    Chapter 1   Introduction Why Are We Ill? xv

Part I..1

    Chapter 2   A City Girl in the Country..3

            Heavenly Mother from Hell.......................................4

            My Shy, Yet Eloquent, Father....................................6

            Byron the Punster...8

            Tiny Girl with a Monkey Grin 9

            Farm Life 10

            The *Fumes* of City Life 11

            The Dolls 19

            An Unpredictable *Grandpa*.....................................20

            More about Our Home 21

            Dance in the Living Room..23

            The Roof Garden...29

            Entering a Dark Tunnel 30

            School Days 32

            Nurse Nancy...39

            Dive for Safety 41

    Chapter 3   I've Got a Brand-New Pair of Roller Skates,

            You've Got a Brand-New Key....................................44

            The Antics of *Bonnie and Clyde* 49

            Going My Way 67

    Chapter 4   Spinning 91

            Dream, Dream, Dream … 93

    Chapter 5   Mile-High Hill 116

            The *Plan* 121

            Little House on Twenty-Fourth Street 131

Faith Is the Bird..138

As It Happened 139

Part Two...147

Chapter 6   The Walk to Find What Was Missing..........149

Happy, Healthy, and *Holy* 155

The *Magic* of Mind Training 157

Miracles 158

Chapter 7   Happy, Healthy, and Whole...........................163

Chapter 8   Life on Life's Terms 166

The Pleasure of Working...172

Chapter 9   Powerlessness and Unmanageability: *God, Grant Me the Serenity to Accept the Things I Cannot Change* 182

Where My "There" Is:..184

The Courage to Change the Things I Can 187

And the Wisdom to Know the Difference 188

Chapter 10 An Inventory..190

The Grief Process..199

Chapter 11 *Stepping* Forward 200

Another step 205

Spirit as defined by Webster[xi].....................................205

Spirit and My Animals 207

Chapter 12 The Diminishment of Suffering and the Eleventh Step 213

Wheel: Who of us has not been drawn—reeling, barreling— into the twenty-first century? Who among us has found peace and quiet?...215

Chapter 13 Working with Chakras 218

Chapter 14 And the Last Shall Be First..........................222

The Promises 223

On Sponsorship...224

Chapter 15 A *Healed* Healer 226

Chapter 16 Meetings: A Room Full of Mirrors 229

Chapter 17 As I Look Back 232

Chapter 18 Appendix..235

Chronic Pain Anonymous[xix] 235
Half measures avail us nothing. 236
In Closing 237
Endnotes 239

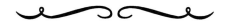

Hello, my name is Sylvia, and I have lived with chronic pain for fifty-eight years. Today I still have the pain, but I no longer suffer. I got my life back. Hurrah, I won, and so can you!

This book tells a little bit of what it was like to live with chronic pain, what happened, and what it is like now. In recovery, this is called experience, strength, and hope. Now I have a fuller and more pleasurable life. I do not mean to upset the apple cart as far as what your beliefs or thoughts might be concerning healing and spirituality, because it is not believing or thinking that really matter. Rather, it is about knowledge, and there can be no question about knowing. I merely ask that you keep an open mind … *for only what is worthy shall I write.*

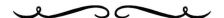

Dedication

I am dedicating this book to Kathleen L. Russell, deceased, who was my devoted counselor in the twelve-step process of recovery from chronic pain. Ms. Russell introduced me to Louise Hay, the words "I am safe," and the firm belief that fear is at the root of dis-ease. She also taught me that by facing this fear head-on, we can conquer it. Kathy, I am sorry you are no longer with us, but in a way you are with me more than ever—I can talk to you now anyplace and anytime. Thank you for all you have taught me.

I need to honor one very faithful friend, Betty Burawski, with whom I attended a chronic pain group back in the nineties. She had an acoustic neuroma removed in 1974. This was a benign growth around the nerve to her left ear which caused her severe headaches and loss of balance. Because there was no laser surgery at the time, she was left almost totally incapacitated from the removal. It took extensive physical rehabilitation to bring her back, but that was only the beginning of her troubles. A cyst was left where the tumor had been and, as a result, it periodically fills with liquid and gives her headaches that often last as long as nine months. We sat together in our misery at those meetings. Betty, I hope you know how much I cherish our friendship.

I would be amiss were I not to mention the saints around us through all this, and they are the spouses and families. I am certain many a time they would like to have said in reference to our contorted faces, "Ah, get over it!" But they didn't. Instead they just stood faithfully by and gave us the time and space we needed to find healing.

Finally, I must not fail to give credit to the people in the rooms of Alcoholics Anonymous, especially those who were with me early on: Diane N., Sondra D., Rachel W., Donna D., Cathy S., Tina H., Beth H. and her husband in sobriety, Fred J. There are countless others, too many to name one-by-one, but we were all gifted with enough desperation to achieve and maintain our sobriety. My first sponsor, Kris K., has made herself available to me now for ten years, and it is to her I owe gratitude for her steady guidance those first, most difficult years. Ruth B., my third sponsor remains a good friend and honorable example—her active listening and deep wisdom have never failed me.

To all these people: I am your teacher and your student as the *miracle* continues to unfold.

Sylvia Deppen

Foreword

I have had the privilege of knowing Sylvia for many years and have known some of her story. However, this book details her story in a very intimate and insightful way. Having come to know her in the later part of her journey, it is a joy to see her recovery and witness how she continues to share her story and help others find pathways to their recoveries. This book is a message of hope and triumph of the human spirit—the healing spirit that exists in everyone that can be realized with the help of others and through *meditation* and *prayer*.

Russ Matthews
Program Supervisor
Behavioral Health
Holy Spirit Hospital
Camp Hill, PA

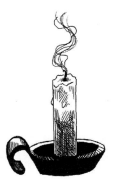

Introduction
Why Are We Ill?

"There is an advantage to bringing nightmares into awareness, but only to teach that they are not real, and that anything they contain is meaningless."[i]

Have you ever wondered why, when two or more people are exposed to similar circumstances—same houses, same bacteria, same nutrition and body types—one person can be stricken by an illness and the other(s) not? I have to also wonder why, when two people are diagnosed with the same illness at the same time, one succumbs quickly and the other stays in good health. The following is an example of this.

There are two women I know who were diagnosed with multiple sclerosis at nearly the same time. One had a family that catered to her every need and demand, and she was soon in a wheelchair requiring help with the most basic of human needs—going to the toilet, taking a bath, and being fed. The other woman, who was the same age, had to work to support her little three-year-old daughter. Today the woman who had things done for her looks like she is at death's doorway, and she sits helplessly waiting to die. She must frequently be totted off to the hospital because of panic attacks, during which she feels she is about to die. The other, who has the three-year-old making constant demands, is still working and has a full life. Why, can you imagine, has one gone downhill so rapidly while the other thrives?

Having found recovery from chronic illness myself in the last ten years, I am questioning the mentality of those who become ill as it relates to that of those who do not. *A Course in Miracles* has helped me to realize that all of life, including our perceived illnesses, is an illusion, and that in reality we are whole and well beings. It is not that our symptoms are not real—not at all—but our perception totally comes into play here.

I have noticed that I seldom become ill anymore. Why is this? Where years ago a cold could take a month to pass, today it will only last a few days at most—that is if I even catch one. The difference, I believe, is my indulgence in mindfulness and meditation. In other words, I keep my thoughts flowing and positive, no longer fixed on problematic thinking. Instead of the thought, "Oh, I'm sick—isn't it awful!" my mind-set is, "Oh, I'm having symptoms, but I will feel better soon." When one's thinking goes in this direction, everything else gets better as well, not just one's health. It has to be that my energy is free and flowing, my chakras unblocked. I feel so blessed.

I recently met a young man with an affliction called multiple sensitivities. He lives a boy in the bubble life—so sheltered. Perfume, cleaning agents and pesticides sprayed on the local crops send him into allergic reactions. He breaks out in rashes and becomes easily nauseated. I feel his depression, too, very deeply. In the brief periods of time I have had to speak with him, mostly because he is either too tired or sick to do so, I have told him how meditation can help him get in touch with deeply rooted, unconscious fears, and how doing so myself is how I finally healed. I tried to emphasize the fact that symptoms and illnesses are very, *very* real—just the permanency of the disease is not. Still, he rebuffs me. I have had to ask myself, "What holds him back from healing?"

For one thing, he is probably surrounded by too many enablers, the biggest of whom is his mother. My prayer for her son is that someday he is allowed enough space—time away from her—to let him adjust his self-image and decide for himself the direction of his life. Another thing is that his mother is an evangelical Christian and probably brought him up in a home where the suffering of Christ on the cross planted in him the idea that he is a miserable sinner. I know this never helped me in my suffering. I am so glad I finally invested in *A Course in Miracles* to sway my thoughts, because I learned that all of life is about a kind of forgiveness, the Creator's, of which none of us are devoid. This realization is what finally heals. It's okay the young man rebuffed me, because someday he'll see I was not judging him. Rather, I was seeing him as he really is: whole.

While with this young man I am also with my elderly aunt who suffers from an ongoing depression. I must be unusually sensitive to these situations because they cause me great sadness. But in departing from the arena of dis-ease I am reminded to be a *healed healer,* and that the reason I was put into such circumstances was to learn one lesson: forgiveness.

I thank God and the many spirits that comprise Him for the ability to see through the sadness around me. I constantly have to remind myself that it is all an illusion—as the course puts it, "Everything is an idea."[ii] Everything is an illusion from which my fellow humans will someday awaken and see themselves in the perfect light by which the Creator sees them. Ah, yes, the light— one does not have to be a character in the television series *The Ghost Whisperer* to see it. We can walk in it all the time by merely turning away from any perceived darkness.

I have wrapped my life up in these few pages. But more than the story of my life, it is the key to becoming a healthier, happier person. If there is only one person out there who I will have helped by writing this, it will have been worth it. Love, fullness of living, and wellness are all there really is; the rest is pure fiction. Please, find this truth in your life too. Be happy, healthy, and whole. It is the only way to be.

PART I

For now we see through a glass darkly ...

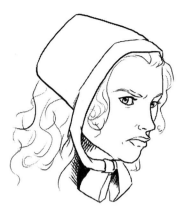

CHAPTER 1

A City Girl in the Country

Wheel: Who of us has not been drawn—reeling,
barreling—into the twenty-first century? Who
among us has found peace and quiet?

*Wheel going around and around, clicking, spinning, driving
me further into life, away from, toward. Where have I
begun, where have I been, and where am I going? I just keep
pedaling around and around … I saw what I saw, I see
what I see, and I will see what there is to see. Oh, wheel going
around and around, clicking, spinning, driving me further,
further, further … When I stop, nobody knows; where I stop,
I know not either. I just am, I just am, I … just … am …
I … am … I … am … I … I … I … am … am … am …*

Since I was a young girl of twelve, growing up on my grandparents'
farm outside Carlisle, Pennsylvania, I have grown accustomed to the
steady roll of bicycle wheels beneath me. My brother and I—sometimes just
myself—would ride out of the city of Harrisburg to the marvelous quiet of

3

the country. Who else but the children of driven business folks, like our parents, would have the inner drive to ride those gruesome seventeen miles of country hills—up, down, up, down? We were all driven people: Mother, Father, Brother Byron, and me, Sylvia. My sister, Wendy, came along years later as a kind of surprise package to our dear, tormented mother, for she was often overwhelmed by the rigors of raising a family and running a business. Yes, the business—photofinishing and cameras—was our father's kind of baby. For over forty-five years, it grew and grew, until it was almost too much for the both of them.

HEAVENLY MOTHER FROM HELL

Mother, I believe, suffered the most. She would try to mother the employees. The dear woman seemed to have no personal boundaries. If an employee was having a hard time at home that a financial boost of advance pay that Father occasionally offered would not remedy, she did her best to find him or her the kind of help needed. She was, indeed, a self-made social worker. Years later, when I started giving my parents more and more problems, she grew to become my social worker too. I was a troubled child, and she was going to find help for me.

Trouble? Yes, I was known as this beginning in my early teens, and I grew worse as an adolescent. It became very apparent when I got even older and had a daughter of my own. The older I got, the more I blamed Mother for all my problems: *It's all your fault, Mother!* Even though I did not say this out loud, I screamed it on the inside. She was, indeed, a responsible business person and commanded respect from her employees. She showed them compassion, and they usually returned her gestures of kindness with thanks. She was so caring. But when it came to being a mother, she admitted, "I just don't know how to be a mother."

There were two aspects of my life she thoroughly encouraged. One was my singing. In third grade, she solicited our Melrose Elementary School music teacher, Miss Malon, to come to our home and give me voice lessons. I remember her telling this lovely young lady, who had blonde, wavy hair to her shoulders and shapely hips under a tight skirt, how I was always swinging and singing like a little bird out on our roof garden. Those were very peaceful and personal times for me—a time to be by myself and only myself. But quite honestly, I did not want to sing for anyone else. I was encouraged to sing in the church choir. Years later, I sang mostly at weddings and at a few funerals. An incident when I was six years old should have been the end to me performing for the public.

We were members of the Methodist church up the street, and one Easter, Mother volunteered me to sing and play my little autoharp. It was my first public performance, and I can remember not being very happy about it. I was so nervous I bit my fingernails to the quick. Mother had me do the piece for her several times before she thought I might be ready. Then there I sat on a small wooden chair, harp on my lap on the rise of our sanctuary. The words to "Rock of Ages"—only three of them—were uttered on key, and I played two chords on the harp. Then, as if on some cue from heaven, I stopped. I froze. I sat there in utter, ghastly silence. Neither words nor chords came to me. Not only was I totally embarrassed, but Father also took me by the hand the whole way home, uttering, "Never again, never again," over and over.

For years as I grew up and sang at all those weddings, I blamed this little fiasco for my inability to put words with the proper notes of music. I struggled and struggled to live up to this ideal. But I couldn't; I just couldn't. Not only that, but when I was with the choir Sunday mornings, I was also the one person in the bunch who would process in and out like a lost duckling. I would invariably go up the wrong aisle or in the wrong direction. This again brought me such grief and embarrassment. I don't know how I ever got in front of an audience again. What was wrong with me? All the other kids seemed to get it right. Many a choir director would shake his or her head in disbelief at my blunders.

Another thing Mother encouraged in me was writing. Again in third grade, we were to write a personal diary. I remember sitting at my small wooden secretary and pouring thoughts out onto paper. Mother was a writer of children's books. She was, however, frustrated in her endeavors to get her books published, but she did manage to get one book published, twice: a Golden Book titled *How to Tell Time in Rhyme*. Many years later, she struggled to get another book, *How to Do Times Tables in Rhyme*, on store shelves and in schools. This latter book got her in some trouble.

Our daughter was in fourth grade and learning the times tables, and Mother brought her new, unpublished book to the school. Apparently she was approaching some of the teachers during school hours about using the book. They were politely trying to tell her, "We're not interested." Finally, the principal called me to ask, "Mrs. Deppen, would you please get your mother to stop coming into our school? We just don't need her book." I felt embarrassed for her and tried to dissuade her actions. It finally must have taken because I heard nothing further from the school.

This kind of friendly persuasion was typical of Mother. When she had an idea, you were expected to at least listen attentively. She would eventually drive that idea home, like a hammer on a nail. She could be, really, all business. That was Millie Hawthorn, my mother. I detested the way she would always come to school to talk to my principal or teachers. I didn't see other mothers doing this. I would have much preferred that she hadn't and had allowed me my own space. I was particularly embarrassed by my fifth-grade teacher, Mrs. Krohl, because she had a tendency to make negative comments about us when we were absent, as if we were malingering.

I like the business finesse Mother left me with and the ability to see my work through to the finish. The difficulty was her inability to be, quite simply, a person. She always said, "I don't like to talk about myself." There was definitely a woundedness about her. She made it clear to me that I was not to talk about myself either. The word "I" was not to come up in a conversation. Now, this could be a good character trait—to a point. Over the years, however, I leaned toward becoming a "nonperson" inside. I believe this is part of why I became so depressed at the ripe young age of ten. I definitely had a wounded side to me too, and I feel not talking about it crippled me for years.

God bless you, Mother, wherever you are. I love you. *I really do.*

MY SHY, YET ELOQUENT, FATHER

My father, known as Dick Hawthorn to most, was a quiet person as opposed to my more persuasive, controlling mother. In retrospect, I really wish he could have discouraged some of her endeavors outside our home. I missed having a mother. Had someone been watching me at the tender age of six, I would not have gotten myself into the trouble that overcame me in later life.

When it came to family time, as we sat at the dinner table, Father could really tell an interesting yarn. He spoke most often of growing up with his father, Dad Hawthorn, and the many business ventures he saw fail for him. Dad Hawthorn was never much for sticking with an endeavor until it came to completion, or at the very least bore any fruit. He spoke most of his trucking, because my grandfather turned one vehicle from a truck to a bus and then back to a truck again over and over. It was all about opportunity. For most of Father's young years, his family had at least the basics, but they certainly did not roll in dough either—not ever.

In the early 1900s, anything with an engine fascinated my Grandfather Hawthorn. At one time he had a potato chip factory, then a confectionary, then an ice cream shop, and often a stall or two at local farmers' markets. Evidently, his mother and my grandmother, Malinda, who grew up on a farm, was not too keen on city life, nor was she keen on his frequently unsuccessful ventures. I understood he could throw some real tantrums, but for the years I knew him—especially in the same house as my mother—he was quite humble. He could get nasty at times, especially when Mother made him take a bath, but mostly he stayed to himself and his room. He always seemed sad to me. I realize more today that he was probably in a lot of pain from having been burned to within an inch of his life from a gasoline fire in one of a number of garages he had.

The fire was caused by confusing gasoline with kerosene. Dad Hawthorn and a good friend were experimenting and trying to create a better rubber for tires when the mistake occurred. They were rushed to Harrisburg Hospital, only to be shoved to the side of a hall on a gurney because they had no medical insurance. No, treatment was not mandatory if you had no money. He had to have suffered horribly. Finally, Malinda and an uncle stormed the hospital and took Dad Hawthorn home, where they somehow got him back on his feet, but I am sure only after months of excruciating pain. He probably got nothing more than a couple of aspirins, if even that. The fact that he was such a frustrated inventor combined with the residual pain from this accident is no doubt the reason we so often heard him in his room saying, "Eiii, eiii, eiii, eiii …" I'm sorry to say we may have even mocked him as children. Today I feel for him, but back then he must have felt so alone in his suffering.

Father's parents grew bitter in the end, and my grandmother went back to her family farm where life was at least a little more predictable, and no doubt more peaceful, too. City life certainly wasn't, I can tell you that.

Father loved the rigors of owning a business and operating a photofinishing plant. He would smile between sighs of fatigue, even when "his baby," the *busyness*, grew bigger than even he expected. My father learned from his father's mistake the benefits of sticking with one good idea and not bouncing from inspiration to inspiration. Machines always broke down, and employees would not always meet Father's expectations, but he loved it. He was kind to everyone too in spite of his often-stressed state when the business grew bigger and bigger and bigger.

If one of the delivery "boys," as they called them, failed to deliver a package to a dealer, Father loved just to take off in one of a number of delivery cars and deliver it personally. He would go as far as Lancaster or Gettysburg. On occasion he traveled to Rochester, New York, to talk with the people who manufactured photo paper at Eastman Kodak. As I said before, as kids we were seldom bored.

Byron the Punster

Growing up in the busyness was fun, for the most part, and those delivery boys often felt like brothers or uncles to me. My real brother, though, was always the most interesting to hear speak. He was an intelligent, fluent punster from our teenage years on up. I hate to admit that during my final years at home before I moved to Florida, I did not appreciate his fun talk. In fact, I hated it! The older and more miserable inside I got, the less I appreciated him. Just like most brothers and sisters, we would have little skirmishes but nothing major. I just had trouble tolerating too much talk. My mother's control issues were problem enough for me, but when the two of them were together, I could not get away soon enough. It would make me feel all the more unable to have thoughts and opinions—wise ones—on my own.

Byron grew to be a tremendous pianist after years of practice. At least to me he was. He could just sit there and touch those keys with such ease, and the sound was so entertaining. I wanted desperately to learn to play too but could not quite master this discipline. He always seemed to show me up; in other words, he just played naturally. I got so frustrated at one point I slammed the keyboard cover down on his knuckles. This is one more thing I was not proud of. I really did like him to play, but as I got older, I got less and less tolerant so that even pleasant sounds were downright annoying. I remember thinking he sounded more like a player piano than a live artist. I could not wait to get out of there.

He is still at it with the puns, taking simple words and bringing a chuckle from all of us. And just as Father would share more at mealtime, so did my brother. Yes, dinner was an interesting and fun time. It was Byron who first taught me the delivery route to the Capitol vendors. It was a precious time riding home on the city bus line together. In the fall, when the sun went down early, we could make faces at each other in the dark reflection of the bus windows. We had many a happy trip rolling through Harrisburg on wheels, wonderfully motor-driven *wheels*.

TINY GIRL WITH A MONKEY GRIN

My sister, Wendy, came along when I was seven and in first grade. She was barely a five-pound bundle and such a little doll for me—a live one. I would pick her up like one of my doll babies, but with the greatest of care so as not to break her. Of course, with the business Mother was delighted I pitched right in to help, but soon her health would begin to hamper things. Having that third child put her over the edge. In the middle of the night, when we were all sound asleep in our bedroom suite out back, I heard Mother scream, "Oh, help me, help me!" Then there was a heavy thud. I went shivering into our parents' room, my bare feet on the cold, smooth wood floor.

"Mother, are you all right?" I cried.

She sat, bewildered, by the side of the bed, Father by now at her side, his hand supporting her back as we all calmed and soothed her. Not until the next morning did we see the damage. Her face was black and blue, and her mouth had a scab on the side where she had been bleeding from biting her tongue. She looked like she had been in an awful brawl, but no one knew what had really happened.

This began a progression of years when she saw doctor after doctor. She was diagnosed with night epilepsy, and she had these nighttime fits only when she got too involved with people or did too much driving. Truly, the rigors of a business and three children were too much for her. She never quite knew where to draw the line between business, family, and her personal life. She had no time for herself. When the stress got to be too much, she retreated many times to the bedroom, and I would hear her in there crying as I stood there wishing I could help. I couldn't.

In the meantime, I did everything I could to help: the laundry and cleaning and caring for Wendy. For a little girl, Wendy was a handful, and I felt confused as to what to do for her. I only wanted to do what was right. I remember her acting out as a four- and five-year-old, screaming at the top of her lungs for what seemed like absolutely no reason. I would try spanking her with all my might, only to have her laugh and scream louder. But her monkey grin—well, it was just downright entertaining, better than Ed Sullivan on television.

To this day I regret having left her home when my brother and I both went off to college. Here again, Mother put herself out for the world of Father, her employees, potential publishers of her children's books, and her many causes over the years. If only she could have drawn a line. Eventually her blood pressure got so high that it destroyed a heart valve. She died too young, but not before leaving a legacy and a footprint of human service. All she wanted to do was help people, and she did.

As for Wendy, she was the toughest little girl—a "mighty mite." She survived. We all did. And I like to think we took on Mother and Father's best character traits. They loved us, and that is all that mattered.

FARM LIFE

When life got too stressful for Mother and Father—for me just too noisy and distracting—we kids would sometimes mount our trusty "steeds," good ole one-speed American bicycles, and ride the seventeen miles to our grandparents' farm. We sometimes went by Williams Grove Speedway and Amusement Park, the last few endless hills going on seemingly forever. And when we finally huffed and puffed into Grandma's sweet-smelling kitchen, fragrant from all the canning and pie and cookie-making, Grandma would swipe a strand of ornery long, grey hair out of her face, smile, and say, "Oh, did you decide to ride your *wheel* all the way up here?"

Ha, as if she didn't know! In her day bicycles were mostly one big wheel. We would laugh at her while digging our hands into the cookie jar. I always hoped for a big, fat, soft sugar cookie.

Today, fifty years later, I still ride my *wheel*. But more than ever before, I ride it with conviction. I see the bicycle as a mode of transportation I wish everyone used more. I wonder if a bicycle isn't today's aerobic substitute for rugged agrarian life. Why do we drive those two-ton vehicles all over creation to get us everywhere we think we need to be? Our bodies have grown grotesquely big and out of shape. The very cars we drive are driving us out of the real world and into a world of hurry up and get there. We have so little sense of where we have been or who we have passed in the process.

Today I rode from our home in Penbrook, outside the city of Harrisburg in central Pennsylvania, ten-miles down to my daughter's home in Middletown. Yes, it is a long way. And there is one very big hill coming home, but my, *my* do I feel alive! And getting there? The joy of arriving is beyond words. I got there on my own steam. I did not pollute this world one bit. I want to give my granddaughters a clean, wholesome place to live, full of promise and where Mother Nature is not violated. I need them to be able to ride where there is clean air and streams running with fresh water. Will they, too, some day ride to the country? Will they experience the earth the way I have? Will they feel it in its purity, and will they ride their wheels freely? Oh, God, I hope so. *Oh, God, I hope so.*

Little did I realize back in the day why riding a bicycle was so refreshing, so therapeutic to me. That would come only after many years of struggle. But a wheel is also a very practical instrument. I pride myself on being in my sixties and still able to take the toughest hill in one burst. Oh, how I want others to experience the exhilaration of riding these Pennsylvania hills, enjoying not just the downhill but also going up … up … up … Because going down is such a pleasure then, one I actually earned.

The *Fumes* of City Life

My earliest perception in life is of being in a big black, shrouded old baby buggy in the den of our house in the city and crying out for Mother. Where was she? I heard her speaking in the next room. As just an infant, I was oblivious about what they spoke of—just grown-up words about, probably the birthing of their real baby, Fine Art Photo and Camera Shop. I don't know where my brother was. He was only about three years old. A later recollection is of sitting with my Grandfather Hawthorn. He was called Dad for all the years I knew him. We were sitting on his lap in a big blue, cushioned, vinyl rocker. I felt so loved and safe there.

At another time I remember lying in my varnished maple crib with a blue teddy bear painted on the headboard. The crib was in a very long room with no window on one of the lower levels of our city apartment. Our quarters were six levels, stretching from Thompson Ally in the back to Derry Street in the front. There were no windows in this room. Why I recall lying there might be that I wanted to touch myself but had been told, "Don't touch yourself *down there!*"

Was this the beginning of my inhibition to feel? Probably not. There is a big, big gap in my memory here. I can tell you the interesting parts of my life in this big edifice of a city building on a city block spanning nearly a quarter of a mile. There was a drugstore on the corner of Nineteenth and Derry Streets, a Laundromat, an appliance store, a barber shop, the entrance to the six-story tenement that contained all the businesses on the lower level, a restaurant, a bar right next to us, and the grey, five-foot wooden gate that entered into our property. Stretching down the hill from us was a beauty salon, two offices with glass show windows, another smaller apartment building, a realtor, and a number of other establishments, the likes of which we would breeze by on our roller skates. Then there was Stine's Grocery Store where we were often sent for a loaf of bread or a quarter pound of Lebanon baloney. I loved when I had an extra penny for a piece of Double Bubble—pink and juicy—which could be blown to the size of your face and then pop! On the end of the block, next to Stine's, was a red-brick apartment building, housing only four apartments.

To say this was an interesting part of town would be a gross understatement, for our lives were beautifully entertained. We had things and people in our lives of which other children could only dream. The bowels of our establishment consisted of a number of rooms darkened to create sharp images on photo paper. To us, however, it meant on off days being able to take our friends through a "fun house," a place filled with spooks and fantasy. Above, where we played during work days, was a roof garden—a *fantastic* roof garden!

Doc Goodyear's pharmacy, confectionary, and drugstore at one end was the center of neighborhood gossip. If you wanted to find out about the locals, you could sit at the soda fountain sipping a five-cent Coca Cola and just listen. Mother's favorite was a cherry Coke with lots of ice. She always liked the ice. Sodas were served in six-ounce waxed cardboard Dixie cups.

Or you could order an ice cream soda, any flavor, served in a tall cut glass with a long spoon and straw. Oh, what a pleasure those times were when Brother and I would sit at the counter, making faces in the huge mirror behind the fountain.

Goodyear's drug store was contained, like the other businesses, at this end of the block by a building they called the Flatiron, mostly because it was in the shape of the base so many women used back then to place the hot iron while pressing their clothes. But oh, the memories I had of that building. I always remember it being so old and creaky. The older it got, the more of a tinderbox it was. I think everyone was afraid of a fire in it. The building we lived in was right up against its red brick walls. We were so close we could hear conversations going on in the various apartments nearest to us. I had a friend named Robert Wentz who lived at the other end on the sixth floor. In the fourth, fifth, and sixth grades, Bobby came to be one of my best friends. He and I would run home together at lunch and after school. He was always faster; he ran like lightning.

I recall the old wooden floors of Doc Goodyear's establishment, but an even homier place for me was right next door to it at the Laundromat. Gerty and Ruth were always there doing people's washing, drying, and ironing. They welcomed our presence as we sat just inside the huge pane-glass window on old grey vinyl-covered chairs and sniffed the clean sent of detergent wrapped in the warmth of the heat given off from the dryers. On a cold winter day, it felt like summer in there, and the windows would fog up with condensation. The floor was covered with black linoleum, often thick with old wax.

Life along a city street can be brutal. There are no bright green lawns or expansive trees, at least where we were. Instead, there was asphalt and people being hit by cars. And cats or squirrels lay dead or dying in the streets. One old white cat, Sparky, hung around our house for years. He eventually became one-eyed from an alley fight. Later I would bring cats back from the country after visiting my grandparents, only to have them smashed in the street. Finally, after about the third or fourth cat, my father saw me boohooing over the loss of another cat and said to me, "Now, Sylvia, you knew this was going to happen." He was right, but his words certainly did not console me.

I'd be amiss if I did not mention the concrete sidewalks outside the businesses on our street. They were eight feet across, seamed slabs of cement.

We appreciated when people kept them smooth for roller skating, but we could not resist putting our initials in newly poured cement. We could skate all the way from Doc Goodyear's to Stein's Grocery. Sometimes if I had a friend with me and only one pair of roller skates, we would share them. It was surprising how easily a single skate could get you from one end of the block to the other.

I recall one instance when my friend Jeanie and I were sharing skates—and this may have been a bit of an omen too. We were on the downhill span between the realtor's office and the grocery store. Jeanie was on one skate and I was on the other. I knew the cement in front of Stein's Grocery was quite rough, so I called out to her, "Jeanie, be careful!" The words were no sooner out of my mouth when I went down, bloodying my knees. I would have best heeded my own warning, do you think?

Next to the Laundromat was Jones's Washing Machine and Appliance Store. Mr. Jones was not one of the friendlier proprietors, but I remember we bought our first Motorola black-and-white television from him. Not long after this, I found it interesting on Sunday evenings. Disney was on the televisions we heard blaring from the windows of our close neighbors in the Flatiron Building. Everybody, it seemed, listened to Walt Disney's charming voice come over that magical box, bringing us the Sorcerer's Apprentice with the biggest celebrity of all times, Mickey Mouse. Saturday mornings, instead of listening to Big John and Sparky on the radio, we would watch *The Lone Ranger* or Roy Rogers and Dale Evens, the greatest cowboys of all times. Father would kid us about the Lone Ranger, whooping, "Hi ho Silver away …" as he waltzed through the room. Silver was the ranger's beautiful white horse. Other times Father would kid, "Everybody knows the good guys who wear the white hats always win."

"Oh, Daddy," we would scold, "don't spoil the suspense!" All the while you could hear fists cracking against faces. He was probably right too; the good guys always did win.

Both cowboys became my secret flames—secret, that is, until my friend Joanne shared her throbbing heart with me. We used to argue when we played house, who would be Roy and who would be Dale? We both wanted to be married to our hero, Roy Rogers. Or who would be rescued by the man in the black mask? Another favorite, and one of my earliest memories of black-and-white television, was Howdy Doody, a marionette, with cantankerous old Mr. Bluster, the red bulb-nosed clown, Clarabelle, who had no strings, and the star himself, Howdy. Looking back, Howdy reminds me a lot of my wiry friend with freckles, Robert, from the tenement next door—plus the strings, that is.

Down from Jones's Appliance was Bob Holmes's barbershop, where Father, Dad, and Brother all got their hair cut. Mother even took me there once or twice to get my hair cut. Oh, how I would protest, "But Mom, I'm not a boy!" She took me there because it was cheaper than the salon where she had hers done weekly. Mother had no creativity in mind when she took me there. How embarrassing! The irony was a beauty salon was for a long time right in the front of the very property where we lived. As a five-year-old I recall slipping into the salon on a Saturday morning and persuading Grace to put red polish on my fingernails, only to have Mother make her take it right off. She'd insist, "Little girls are not supposed to wear red nail polish or lipstick!" Red seemed to be about the only color they had back then.

Next to the barbershop was the entrance to the six-story tenement. Inside the ten-foot-high doors with a glass transom bearing the numbers 1911 was a wide staircase leading up to the second floor. I seldom ventured up those creaky stairs. From what I recall, they were just wood and probably termite-eaten underneath. I hated going up there. Mother sometimes sent me up them to inquire of a neighbor as to their health. I think really she wanted to know if a woman and her children had survived the argument she heard from one of the windows left open on a hot summer day. Living with these people next door got to be a bit of a soap opera day-by-day. Mother was so sensitive to people's struggles, especially the women.

On the second floor was a musty, old, high-ceiling ballroom where the upper class once had extravagant dances. The few times I got to stroll and cartwheel through it, it was only filled with musty crates and cardboard boxes of junk. It held remnants, no doubt, of the many lives that occupied that gossamer building. Bobby at times would tell me about some of the many interesting people, his neighbors, who lived there. I do wish in hindsight that I had asked him more about his life because years later I began to know him better—more deeply, sadly—but only after much time had passed between us. I later realized he was a very isolated person and had never known his father. His mother protected him almost beyond reason. I remember her shaking him, scolding him, and needing to know every place he had been and with whom he had been. But between us at this time there was only joy and fleeting companionship. I would not realize until many years later that his speed in running was a symptom of a *dis-ease* he and I both acquired: alcoholism. But it had yet to touch us at this young age.

A lower floor held the office of our dentist, who I swear did not know what Novocain was, because I remember him pulling a tooth with one big yank! Dr. Cortalazi was the only dentist I knew back then. Years later I disrespectfully referred to him as Dr. Corta-*lousy*. My brother was sensible enough to ask for Dr. Bailey down the street. I came to eventually judge myself devoid of common sense since I was born on April Fool's Day. How else could I explain the kind of dizzying sense of *"Are you just that dumb?"* It was a question not only heard of me but also said by me to find out why I made sooo … many seemingly stupid decisions. Was I dumb? Am I dumb? I will let you decide … Maybe life just sent me too many puzzling questions. I didn't know—not back then. Today the answer is easy, but in the '50s, '60s, '70s, '80s, and even through most of the '90s, I was truly *dumb*founded.

Next to the stairway up to the tenement, a kind of Peyton Place, was the high, steamy window to John's Restaurant. Inside, Connie and John would be flipping burgers or shaking the sizzling basket full of French fries. There was a high, pressed metal ceiling where fans cooled satisfied eaters at the long counter. I loved when Dad brought home a tall glass bottle of grape soda pop with two straws. My, how our tongues luxuriated with the zippy carbonated taste. The first sip always brought tears to my eyes. Father's employees frequented this place at lunch time. I always knew where they had been when they came back to work; they smelled like a walking French fry. Just like at Doc Goodyear's, there were tall stools that pivoted under us. And as children, we spun around on them like a carousel at an amusement park—around and around and around we went until our heads felt like they were dangling from the fan above.

Next to John's was the last place before our gate. This place held a lot of mystery in my juvenile brain and a lot of intrigue too, for this was the place we were not to set foot in, under any circumstances. It was a bar—the *den of evil*, as put forth by Mother. Evil did seem to escape into the atmosphere outside its window that opened onto our roof garden, where we so often played. We could hear people talking over the sound of the jukebox. A bar, too, is not a bar unless there is an occasional brawl, and they had brawls. I would sometimes see someone come flying out the front entrance, bounced either by the bartender or the opposing fighter. The struggle sometimes ended up in the street. I know, if she could, Mother would have rather we had not seen such images. But it happened, and we saw it all.

Next came the address 1917 in big black numbers on a grey wooden gate that was scrolled at the top. Yes, this was our house. The heavy black hinges of this gate gave out a scolding, clanking sound upon opening. Inside and down to the left was a metal box labeled "Harrisburg Dairy" and containing empty glass bottles to be picked up by the milkman in the early morning. A long cement walkway led back to a metal stairway leading upstairs to two apartments—the second and third floors. Behind this was the walkway that led to our entrance. My, the living that went on behind this door was such an adventure, so full of intrigue and fantasy. I wonder if I can do it justice in these few short pages, but I will be brief and to the point. I must not miss a thing, for it all forms in my mind a kind of Disneyland and a place my cohorts came to envy over these fun years. Where do I start?

The closet on the left as you would enter was filled with warm coats, jackets, sweaters, gloves, mittens, and hats. Mine was either a knit cap or a little white straw hat with a blue ribbon on it. Mother's was a neat little felt hat with a feather on the side, and a long pin to keep it in place. Father's was the traditional hat for men in those days: felt, broad-brimmed, and with a wide band around the crown.

I can still see my mother's face when she placed that hat on her head—sweet, dimpled, big hazel eyes and bright red lipstick with a tinge of it on her cheeks. She was the more engaging of our parents, always attempting to persuade a person when it came to "ought tos" or "shoulds." Father's face was heavy set, with deep brown eyes. He was quiet and pensive, but he had a captivating way about him when he spoke. He was a storyteller at heart, and he told us many stories, often as we sat around the dinner table. I can see the twinkle in his eyes still as he shared the history of his father, the inventor, Ed Hawthorn. They ended in tragedy but spoke of his ability to create "things"—a potato chip making machine, a motorized cart out of scooter parts, an airplane, a bus that became a truck and then a bus again … and then a truck again, and many other ingenious inventions. That was Dad Hawthorn, my grandfather.

Past the coat closet on the right was our bathroom. A lot of history went on in that room. It had a black tile floor and a white enamel sink with

17

a cupboard below for cleaning supplies, powders, a sponge or rag, and the plumbing. Above it was the medicine closet and the mirror where I was first introduced to myself. Need I mention the toilet? And yes, there was a big lion's-paw bathtub. Saturday mornings were sometimes the most amusing, as Mother insisted Dad Hawthorn "Get a bath!" once a month. Because he hated getting a bath, his words to her were, "Eiii … eiii … eiii … You're right, and the world is wrong! Eiii … eiii … eiii …" Talk about invasion of privacy, but someone had to do it!

On the left, next to the coat closet, was the entrance to what at first was Gra-Mar Beauty Salon, for Grace and Marge. I knew it as the salon when I was little and a place I could observe the efforts of women to get, in Father's words, "beautified." I smelled the pungent odor of wave and perm lotions, and ladies would sit with their hair in pin curls under hot dryer hoods. Years later the salon moved up Derry Street further and our photo outlet and camera store occupied this space.

We had an interesting living room. Father had a stone facade installed on the wall closest to that side entrance. There was an aquarium in that wall with angel fish, a catfish, colorful neons, various other tropical fish, and a snail. I was intrigued by a small treasure chest, the contents of which sparkled with each bubble rising rhythmically from the lid to the surface. Each time the lid would snap back shut and I would anticipate the next bubble. This room would come alive with dancing when Father put Copeland's "Rodeo" music on the cabinet stereo. I loved this composition with the sound of a horse neighing and his hooves clomping. At Christmastime we usually had a large cut evergreen in the corner of the room. Mother and Father made a tradition of decorating it themselves. They would tell us, "Santa wants to decorate it." But I suspect a bit of romance was involved for the two of them.

Business income was up at times and down at times, but we never went without. We were blessed with some pretty wonderful gifts at Christmas. I was once given a walking doll I named Penny. If you put her in a certain position next to you and took her arm in a certain way, her legs would actually move forward, one after the other. And she had what looked like real hair. I was so intrigued by how her hair was so much like my own that I proceeded to wash it and cut it. Oh, the disappointment I felt—it was a real "bad hair day" for Penny, and no one could fix it. Like I suppose it must

18

have been for other girls like me, I imagined my dolls were real. And when a mother cannot fix her "child," it is heart rending. I sensed Mother wanted to *fix* me in later years when she began to sense the kind of desperate and miserable malady I was living. It seemed something was wrong with her child—something no one could fix.

One year Dad Hawthorn got a beautiful doll for my sister, Wendy. Dad could sound awfully gruff and miserable, which he must have been because we commonly heard his "eiii … eiii … eiii … eiii …" resounding throughout the back of the house where his room was. But when my sister responded with such excitement at the sight of this beautiful doll, I saw tears come to his eyes.

I could not believe my ears years later when Wendy told me Mother had made him take the doll back! Now why would she do that? The poor old fellow always seemed so beaten down. Was such a small pleasure too much to expect for him? Did she hate the man that much? I understand her now and why she may have resented such a gesture. I believe the child in her had died when she was quite young, like maybe around the age of ten. Not only that, I think she just plain had it in for the man.

The Dolls

I had a favorite doll when I was an infant and toddler. Her name was Pixie, and she had a darling little face on a kind of plastic head with painted hair. Her body was a soft rubber. I would carefully dress her and undress her in her overalls and blouse or a dress or pajamas. I would either set her in the little wooden play high chair or at the table with a stuffed animal or two for friends. I imagined her to be real, with real feelings and real needs, so I made sure she was fed and happy. I will never forget one day when I was about five.

Apparently the rubber of her body had grown old and cracked, because one day, to my horror, the head fell off her body. I was grief stricken, so Mother took her to a place called "The Doll Hospital." It was on the 1500 block of Derry Street. When they were done with her, Mother took me to pick her up. I wish someone would have gotten a picture of my face when I saw her. Here they had put a new, smaller body on Pixie, one that was too small for her head. Again I was grief stricken. To me, it was not even Pixie anymore.

This may sound a bit austere, but this incident of my "child" losing her head may have been another kind of omen too. What happened surreptitiously the very next year in hindsight was very much like this incident with the doll. My life would never be the same either. This particular incident, much like children will do, remained buried in my psyche for forty-five years. I don't know if this is a bad thing. It may have saved me from being made an invalid early on because I had to struggle to stay on top of it. Otherwise I may have been pampered and coddled, making me weak. Only God knows these things. But I vividly recall another incident that told the story of how wounded I really became.

I was ten years old, right after the clouds of depression descended over my life, and I was lying on the bed in an upstairs bedroom. I had another doll in my arms, a smaller one. As I lay there feeling broken, in my mind I prayed that the doll—this "child" in my arms—might come to life. I believe today that what I really wanted was for my unbroken child to come back to life because I was really feeling broken myself. I lay there hoping, wishing, and praying with all my inner fortitude, for life to come into that doll—me. Somehow I felt if she came alive I would get my life back too. Of course, that doll was just a doll, and I stayed dead inside for a very long time.

AN UNPREDICTABLE GRANDPA

My mother and her older brother and younger sister were raised in the quiet of a Cumberland County farm. Her father, my Grandfather Allen, could be of a peculiar nature. When we played there as children, he could be having a wonderful time, laughing right along with us. Then, out of the blue, his mood would turn dark, and the playful raking of leaves in the fall turned into raking the whole front lawn. It almost seemed like he did not want us to have fun—at least we pouted this under our breath. Years later, my dear Aunt Aileen told me something sad about my mother when she was young.

One day, when Mother was about nine or ten, apparently she had been dancing and skipping through the upstairs rooms of the farmhouse, as little girls do at times. Grandpa must have had one of his moods, because in an effort to quiet and still her, he tied her to the bedstead. This almost sounds too cruel to repeat. However, for one, I believe each of us reflects sometimes in our lives the *sins of our fathers* (i.e., we repeat the trauma inflicted upon us by those who went before us). For this, I am able to forgive such a happening. Years later, another sad story surfaced about my Uncle Stephen, Mother's brother.

Apparently Grandpa Allen had inflicted some such similar punishment upon their eldest child, my Uncle Stephen. Of course, I was not there to know what it was, and I was never told exactly what happened to him. World War II may have affected him too. But I did experience the pain of seeing how the sins of their father were visited upon my cousins in Massachusetts. To this day, it tears my heart out. Sometimes I think to myself, *If only I had known what happened to my cousin, Shelley, and her older sister, Adrienne, maybe I could have helped some.* Shelly became schizophrenic and a street person and disappeared mysteriously for many years. Adrienne led the relatively normal life of a lesbian but always seemed bitter for whatever reason. But we were young together, and such is just speculation on my part. Still, it hurts.

MORE ABOUT OUR HOME

Christmas was a delightful time of year in our house. It was also a stressful time, as Father became oppressed somewhat with needing to get photo Christmas cards out on time for customers. We did not have digital photography, like we do today, so people could not print out their own cards. It was up to Father to see that they were exposed sharply on the paper, cut, neatly packaged, and distributed to various drug stores and the Pennsylvania State Capitol eateries run by blind vendors around our state complex. We didn't have Facebook or e-mail that, when our hearts were ripe with love for family and friends, we could just click and send greetings. Father was conscientious about the work we put out.

I use the word *we* because in the early days of the business, we would sit as children at the "dope tray"—especially my brother and I, because Wendy came along seven years after me as a kind of surprise package. "Dope" was a combination of chemicals that brought the images out of the photo paper. Those sharp black-and-white images were so fascinating—like magic! With rubber gloves to protect our hands, we swished the solution over little four inch-by-four inch or four inch-by-five inch pieces of paper. And voila—people and things, precious faces, scenes, and belongings, appeared, one-by-one, caught for posterity by the eye of a camera. There were even pictures of dead people in caskets at viewings! I would be remiss, at this point, if I did not mention the value a camera held to our parents. Yes, we were kept in business because people took pictures. It was our livelihood. But there was something else.

Mother and Father dated at Camera Club meetings, and a number of their best friends were also members of this club. Before marrying my mother, Father worked for another camera shop and photofinisher named Lett's. Later, Mother and Father opened their own business, Fine Art Photo, with an artist's palette for their logo. Customers drove up and parked in Thompson Alley in the back at first. As a four-year-old, I was often the official greeter because I loved when someone gave me a lift onto the counter of their Dutch door so I could charm and be charmed by customers.

One of my mother's winning photos was an eight-inch by ten-inch, black-and-white matted photo of my beloved Aunt Aileen, standing out at the mailbox at home on their Carlisle farm. She was a beauty (and still is at eighty-seven-years old). It was displayed either in the window of our camera shop that eventually took the place of the hair salon in the front of our property or in a gold frame around our city apartment, along with other spectacular snapshots. Some were displayed in the showcase windows of dealerships like Rea & Derrick's drugstores or Kaplan's Pharmacy on the Square in Harrisburg. Images of our growing up accompanied them, because Mother kept a camera close at hand around the house. One rather embarrassing one is of me, only a year old, with a pixie grin on my face and my butt stuck down in a white, porcelain chamber pot. These photos were a source of great pride for Mother—my own pride too because I could feel hers. The photos led to a lot of chuckling when company came.

Our first kitchen was tiny and situated off the dining room. I remember many a morning dipping our buttered toast into Dad's sweet, milky coffee. As ornery as the old man could be, it did not scare us—we loved him. Or at least I did. He was the one member of the family I could count on being around and not busy all the time. I remember him papering that dining room with a leafy green paper. Our table, which sits empty today in my basement, was maple and had two leaf extensions. Dad often sat leaning his elbows on the table. We were afraid the extension would give way, sending his dinner, his drink, and any other dish thereon onto his lap and the floor. I recall it did collapse once. Byron, Mother, Father, and I would sing, "Dad Hawthorn, if you're able, get your elbows off the table." His response was, "Eii … eii … eii … eii …" with a chuckle and a twinkle in his eye.

Wendy was pretty young still, and Mother worried she was not eating enough. We played "airplane into the hangar." The food on the spoon was the airplane, and her mouth was the hangar. It was an effective game that Dr. Klitch warned might someday fatten her up a little too much, and it did—a little.

Dance in the Living Room

We had hardwood, oak floors throughout our place, and often my Grandmother Allen's carpets would be thrown on top. I loved her braided rag-rug carpets because I could pick out the different outfits I had worn growing up. There was the green wool of an old coat I wore at the age of five, the blue denim of an old pair of Grandpa's workpants, and a pink-and-white light cotton dress I wore to my friend Judy's sixth birthday party. She even included some of my sister's baptism dress, a bit of white fluff in the midst of the other heavier fabrics. Those carpets practically told the story of our growing up on the farm and in the city. Years later we actually had a fancy store-bought grey woolen carpet laid throughout the main rooms.

Right behind that stone facade was a big closet and dressing room where we hung most of the outfits my sister and I wore. In the early years, our bedrooms were actually detached from the main house, separated by a roof garden. But for now we would dress here, gazing at the results in a mirror attached to the back of the closet door. I kept my petticoats stored here too because my favorite thing was just to dress in a petticoat or two or three … whatever it took to send me spinning out into the living room area where I could dance for Father. My, could I spin and dance! I saw his face, as tired as he often was, just light up to see me dancing just for him. In my child brain, I was a ballerina at Radio City Music Hall where Mother sometimes took us in New York City. Over the years she would take us there on occasion as she attempted to get her children's books published.

The wall opposite the stone facade was rather plainly papered, but it had a window in it. This window did not look to the outside like a normal window. Rather, it looked out over a staircase that went down to the shop below. But that wall was papered with a lovely vine-over-trellis design. My mother liked things to at least look natural. She didn't like that we lived in the city, and she did her best to bring at least the illusion of country into our home. That is why from an early age we children were sent frequently to experience the farm where she grew up in Carlisle, Cumberland County.

I recall the old Motorola television cabinet sitting right below this illusive window. I was fascinated once when the repairman took the guts out of it to take to the shop for repairs. My brother and I took turns getting inside the cabinet and pretending we were Uncle Bob or the Indian Princess Winterspringsummerfall—Howdy Doody's cohorts—performing for all the world to see. We were stars in our own right!

At one point I had a moderate-size wooden desk on the inner wall of this room. It was in a recessed area. I can still see the little rubber eraser, wooden ruler, pencils, and goose-necked lamp. I smell the pungent shavings from the pencil sharpener. It felt so private, and I was comfortable there with my thoughts. Who cared there was homework spread out in front of me? I had some pretty deep thinking to do.

I remember one evening when I had my friend Donna Rolleston there for supper. Mother could not get done reminding me I had homework to do! So I sat at the desk trying to concentrate, knowing all the while I had a friend there. I think I tried to entertain her with some books—I guess she did not have homework—but she kept interrupting my concentration. I told her abruptly, "You have to go home now!" She got so insulted, like I did not want her there, which I really did. It must have been the way I said it that was insulting. I was only mimicking Mother's behavior when we were underfoot and she needed to focus on the business. If Donna were here today, I would apologize to her.

The green vinyl couch and Father's old easy chair were on the outside wall. When I was still quite little, I would go behind him in his chair and run my fingers back and forth over his scalp, as if I were Grace or Marge in the old beauty shop shampooing his hair. I would go, "Shampoo, shampoo, shampoo …" It must have given him great pleasure, just as it brings to mind the wonderful intimacy I felt with him. It was an intimacy, I am afraid, that in years to come would dwindle. His "baby," the business, grew out of proportion, stressing him more and more. His heart was getting the worst of it in ways we did not realize. For many years he and Jim Knaub mixed huge vats of chemicals for color processing—Father was proud to have the first color lab in our town—but they did not know to wear masks to protect their lungs from the strong odors given off from this process. In the end, this is what left him fighting for his life.

The very back room, right next to the roof garden, was a den for a long time. This is where that black, shrouded baby buggy once sat, and my little ears were perched listening for Mother's voice. And this, too, is where that big, overstuffed rocker was when Dad had Byron and me, only infants, on his lap. Oh, the feelings of warmth, love, and security I got there. It planted a sense of wellbeing in me, the kind I would draw on in the turbulent years that were to follow. Mother and Dad Hawthorn were mostly at odds, but I am sure, now that they are both gone to the next life, my mother realizes just how much he gave me by holding me and loving me. I needed that time with this frustrated inventor of a grandfather, because, I feel now, he planted a kind of treasure in such a little tike. I would come to need a lot of physical and moral strength. The life I faced would do me so much injustice, that in looking back, I am in awe of how I ever made it. I should have died. Did I cheat death? Or was it just not my time to die? That part of my story is coming. Maybe you can help me learn the answer.

Next to our little dining room was a set of stairs that led to the shop below and where my bedroom had once been. We moved around and changed our living areas so frequently that just about every room had multiple purposes over the years. But it was this particular staircase that would wreak havoc on my life. I will not say more about this now. But yes, these are the infamous stairs I managed to put out of my mind for the better part of a lifetime. What happened remained buried in my psyche. I unknowingly stuffed it like children often do.

Eventually, that den in the back became our new kitchen, modern appliances and all. We even had a double stainless steel sink with a sprayer nozzle. One employee, Virginia Booser, was like family because she helped Mother out around the house and with us. She would even wash dishes for us. She was my mentor, my example of how helpful I could be to Mother. I did respect and love Virginia. She was from a good Catholic family of ten children, and she knew what hard work was. She taught me the value of working together. We got the job done when Virginia was around, and she had the nicest way of telling us how to do things—she showed us. I know my mother admired her too.

In later years I sensed Virginia harbored some resentment toward both my parents. I am not sure what this was about, except maybe it had something to do with the hiring and letting go that goes on in any business. They had to let her go at some point. This was sad, but it had nothing to do with anything she had done wrong. We loved her—a lot.

> *Wheel going around and around, clicking, spinning, driving*
> *me further into life, away from, toward. Where have I*
> *begun, where have I been, where am I going? I just keep*
> *pedaling, around and around ... I saw what I saw, I see*
> *what I see, I will see what there is to see. Oh, wheel going*
> *around and around, clicking, spinning, driving me further,*
> *further, further ... When I stop, nobody knows; where I*
> *stop I know not either. I just am, I just am, I ... just ... am.*
> *I ... am ... I am ... I ... I ... I ... am ... am ... am ...*

Life lived around a family business could get pretty confusing. The store was in the front of our building eventually, but there were buzzers and bells all throughout the house to alert us when a customer walked in. There was no such thing as just sitting down to a meal because we would hear the bells going off. And if the store clerk had a question, either Father or Mother or both were called up front over an intercom. Depending on the customer and the issues, a simple meal could get pretty stressful. As an eleven-year–old, I learned to stay out of their way by mounting my sturdy one-speed bicycle, with wide tires and a bell on the handlebars, and riding to the country and into the arms of my waiting grandparents.

Our parents were very, very engaged, hardworking people. Most of the customers and employees held them in high regard, but I have to wonder to what end it brought them. Was it worth it? Father's heart was so bad in the end, and he wanted to live so desperately that he was injecting chemicals into his own heart just to get him through another day. Still, he took great pride in what he was doing. Another passion he had was for reading. His favorite pastime, especially years later after he got sick, was an open book and a big *Webster's Dictionary* nearby.

I recall frequently hearing Mother proclaim proudly how before the photofinishing, he first went into business with his friend Leo Koralik from Chicago. Leo talked him into going along with him and selling *The World Book Encyclopedia*. Father, being the astute businessman he was, decided the best way to do this was to first read the whole set himself. What better way could he speak of what lay between the covers of those awesome books? My mother knew she had married an intelligent man because he would sit at the dinner table or around the living room with guests and spout out facts, details, and timelines like he was reading directly from one of his books.

The old kitchen where we had once dunked toast in coffee with old Dad became his bedroom eventually. A walk throughout the house was musical in that every so many floor boards would creak underfoot. I always sped up when I got close to Dad's room. It had a stringent odor from heavy liniment and body odor. No, Dad did not like to take baths. This and other character traits in him made something else undesirable.

Fine Art Photo sent delivery boys out into the city every afternoon—why they were called "boys" I have no clue because they were grown men! The boys would take packages of finished photos to the various distributors around town, mostly pharmacies. My mother, Millie Hawthorn everyone called her, had a bend for controlling things. She insisted Dad go along on these trips, thus "getting him out of the house." I know those delivery men dreaded sitting next to this foul-smelling old man, who would cuss at the other drivers and send thick projectiles of spit out his window, sometimes missing and hitting the side of the car. Yuck. I believe we lost a few good delivery men this way.

Besides using the off hours to take friends into the inner sanctum of the dark developing rooms downstairs, we had another way of entertaining friends. I would take the hand mirror from the bathroom and whatever other mirrors I could find around the house, and by looking down into the mirror's reflection of the ceiling above, we found ourselves walking on the ceilings throughout the house. I remember feeling like a trapeze artist in the circus, flying through the room. Try it once. You'll see—it's fantastic.

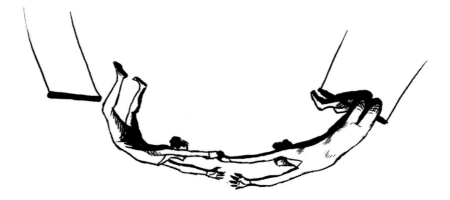

The employee break room was on the lower level at the alley. I enjoyed sitting amongst the employees, watching them drink coffee and smoke. One interesting lady, Vada, demonstrated sending up smoke rings. Another woman, Kitty, would ask me occasionally, "Have you been smoking bonbons and eating cigarettes?" After this she pealed out musical laughter, pulling us all into an altered state of mind. We sat in old maple chairs and couches with foam-stuffed cushions of rough plaid material. Most of the employees were women, except for a few good men. I will never forget George Nissle.

George was young, good looking and single. I could never understand how such a gentle man could stay unmarried so long. For the longest time I never even heard him even speak of a girlfriend. Maybe he was just really private. It was not my business, but I wondered. I even fantasized about being his wife. Once when Mother and Father treated the employees to a boat trip down the Chesapeake Bay, swimming, and a picnic, I saw him with a can of beer in his hand. He seemed so relaxed and happy. Pointing to the beer, I asked Mother, "Can I have one of those?" I was only eleven, and even though we lived next to a bar I was clueless about alcohol. You can guess Mother's response. George did finally marry, years later.

THE ROOF GARDEN

I could devote a whole volume about this next place in our home: the roof garden. I spent many an hour swinging and singing like a canary in this place, situated between the den and our bedrooms in the back. Yes, to go to bed we had to walk outside, wearing coats and boots during inclement weather. Father built a boardwalk to protect the green gravel tar paper roofing from being destroyed by our shoes, and it kept our feet dry when it rained or snowed.

The outer edge of the garden had big, wooden, green-painted, rectangular flower boxes on it. Mother kept these planted with arborvitaes, petunias, geraniums, and marigolds. Her favorite was a box of Lilies of the Valley right by the back kitchen door. There was even an occasional watermelon vine, as a result of our seed-spitting contests. A tub or two of arborvitaes sat at various points on the boardwalk. The far side of the garden had skylights that opened up to provide air to the shop below. Our curious ears would pick up conversations between employees as they worked. When we were little, there was a large rectangular wooden sandbox for us to play in. Father built it, but often we could not use it because the cat liked it too, and it could smell pretty nasty. The metal swing set and slide were also on a boardwalk to the center of the garden. In the summer we put the slide into the nice-size, above-the-roof swimming pool. This created a problem one summer when I was about ten years old.

One of Father's employees, Dottie Wilson, had given my friend Joanne and me some of her old dresses and scarves to use to play dress up. Among the things were two pairs of lovely spiked heels. Maybe you can guess what happened. Joanne and I were tickled that Dottie's shoes were so tiny that they actually fit our little feet. We tromped all over the hot tarpaper roof. That afternoon, we got our bathing suits on and came splashing down the sliding board into the pool. Of course this sent a torrent of water out of the pool and onto Father's roof. We had only been swimming maybe ten minutes when Father came up with an enraged expression on his face. Our spiked heels had left huge holes, and water was dripping down onto the employees' heads below! Well, as you can imagine, that was the end of spiked heels on the roof.

Another incident took place as a result of having an outdoor walkway between the house and the bedrooms. One day my friend Joanne and I put our swimming suits on in the bathroom of the house. We went about swimming. Afterward, mindlessly, we took our suits off in the bedrooms, forgetting our cloths were in the house. So, rather than putting the cold, wet suits back on, we decided to make a naked dash across the roof garden to get to our clothes. To our embarrassment, the upstairs neighbors were sitting out on their porch. We must have made quite a spectacle, because they were laughing their sides off at us.

The inside ledge of the garden was smack up against the red bricks of the Flatiron Building. There was one window into the bar next door. I enjoyed the soft light, music, and muffled voices that came through it on a warm summer evening. We would trudge past it as we went off to bed for the night.

Most of my times on the roof garden were fun: the fashion shows with the skylights as our stage, an old crate on top of one of the skylights with doors and windows cut into it, and listening to laughter and conversation below. We lived idyllic lives. However, from about age eight and up my life seem to take a turn south as I entered a kind of dark tunnel that became my life for forty-three years. Then the roof garden became more of a prison, and the back stairs to the alley were the forbidden exit into the world.

ENTERING A DARK TUNNEL

I recall the very time, day, and place when the veil descended upon my life. I had been visiting my aunt, uncle, and cousin in Waldwich, New Jersey. The day prior I had been embarrassed by a kind of newfound sexuality in my ten-year-old body. The family had gone to a concert that afternoon, leaving my uncle, cousin, and sister at home with me. The three of us girls took a bath together and then went romping skinny-naked throughout the house. My uncle powdered our up-turned bottoms, and this is when I felt wretchedly exposed. I quickly dressed myself and withdrew in embarrassment to one of the bedrooms upstairs. I honestly at the time did not know what happened inside me. But the next day as I came downstairs, a kind of darkness came over me, and it stayed there for thirty-seven miserable years. Yes, I was deeply and mysteriously depressed.

In the meantime, I went on singing, dancing, and playing the fool, as if there was not a problem in the world. The darkness stayed my little secret. However, I must have complained too much to mother, and I believe the words were simply this: "I hurt." Every so often she would haul me off to Dr. Klitch's office with this simple, vague complaint. And invariably, the doctor would say, "It must just be growing pains." I remember thinking to myself, *Well, if it's growing pains, I don't want to grow!*

The bedroom suite had three rooms—the large main room for our parents' big maple bed, the smaller room for my brother, and the smallest for my bed and dolls. We had no bathroom in the back, so we used a small porcelain chamber pot, which I hated to empty when it was my turn. Father and Byron built a railroad yard on a large platform in our parents' room. It was on hinges and could be folded up against the wall when not in use.

My little six-by-eight room felt perfect. It even had a small cedar closet with a trap door situated up high on the wall, over the staircase that led down to the shop and alley. When I was little, I loved to hide in that closet. I could hear conversations downstairs among the employees, and no one knew I was listening. It was a good place to disappear to when we played hide and seek too or when I just needed a place to think. In one corner of the room was a small table where I kept my children fed and entertained. Each doll baby felt real. I would dress them and make up conversations. As the years progressed and Mother and Father became more and more occupied by the business, my family of dolls told me how lonely they were when I was not with them. I began to feel lonely and sick inside too. Then, when I entered that dark tunnel, even sunny days were dark.

> *Wheel going around and around, clicking, spinning, driving*
> *me further into life, away from, toward. Where have I*
> *begun, where have I been, where am I going? I just keep*
> *pedaling, around and around ... I saw what I saw, I see*
> *what I see, I will see what there is to see. Oh, wheel going*
> *around and around, clicking, spinning, driving me further,*
> *further, further ... When I stop, nobody knows; where I*
> *stop I know not either. I just am, I just am, I ... just ... am.*
> *I ... am ... I am ... I ... I ... I ... am ... am ... am ...*

SCHOOL DAYS

In 1954, there was no public kindergarten, so I had to start in the first grade. I had Miss Tanler for the first two years. I remember being so scared on that first day of school. But the teacher quickly dissolved my fears. She was not only kind; she was also fun to be with. I loved the wooden desks and chairs, which we had to carefully line up before recess or going home in the afternoon. I loved the yellow-lined tablets, thick wooden pencils, and boxes of large colored crayons. The teacher had a long pointer she used to point out numbers and letters on a long poster above the blackboard. It delighted me when I was allowed to take the erasers to the playground and bang them together to get the chalk dust off. Everything about those first days of school was exciting.

I began school as a normal child, but by October of that year, things changed for me. The phrase, "I hurt, Mommy," began to come frequently. It perplexed my family. Mostly my face hurt, because I kept wanting to close my eyes to stop the pain. When Miss Tanler had us put our heads down on the desk, the other children protested, but it was comforting to me. Like most children, I had a tendency to daydream. But as the years progressed, I did it more and more as an escape.

In Melrose Elementary, learning and school were new and exciting. Still, by age eight I went to bed at night longing to feel my mother's hand on my brow, comforting me. And she was there for me whenever Father and the business would let go of her. By age ten, when the dark veil first came over me, I began dreaming of my own heroic demise, that I had sacrificed my life for that of another. I dreamed I had been convicted wrongly of some horrible crime and was in jail for it. I don't know why such thoughts occurred to me; they just did. By ages twelve and fourteen, I dreamed I was dying because I felt that way.

Having had Miss Tanler for first and second grades, I wasn't sure I wanted to move on, but my third-grade teacher, Miss Kreider, had long, wavy blonde hair, and she was tall, slender, and a real beauty when she smiled. I looked up at her in awe. Our old Melrose School had no gym, so on nice days we went out to the playground to run. On rainy or snowy days, we went to the musty-smelling unfinished basement. I liked the square dancing because we got to choose partners. I remember one pudgy little guy named Dennis who always picked me for his partner. I had a favorite, too—Dwight Romanovitz. He was in my dreams. I'm afraid he didn't even see me. However, I did get to go to a birthday party at his house.

I had a fear of needles—don't most kids? Even some grown men I know do too. But from first through second grades, we were lined up to get our polio shots. I waited my turn in line, dreading it. I was glad when the next year they finally started to give a palatable liquid that we could drink instead of an injection. I really had no idea what it would have been like had I or anyone I loved gotten polio. This lesson came years later. Miss Kreider had an engagement ring on her finger before the end of the year. Some guy got really lucky.

I was assigned Miss Asper in the fourth grade. I worried all summer. She was a tall, lanky kind of woman with dark features, her legs a jungle of thick, dark hair. However, my fears were quickly gone after the first day. As it turned out, she was very nice. I learned to love reading in her class. Our reader was a brown, cloth-covered book with a covered wagon pulled by oxen on the front called *Wagons West*. This was the year I first met my neighbor and friend, Bobby Wentz. Robert, as I called him, was in the class across the hall. When it was time to go out to get a tray of half-pint milks from the cooler opposite our classroom, I would go slowly by their door hoping to get his attention inside the room and wave. At lunch and after school, Robert raced me home. In fact, most of my memories of him are of racing. He went everywhere fast! I did not realize it at the time, but he had horrible social anxiety.

I had a friend named Judy in Miss Asper's classroom. One day that year Judy did not come back to school after lunch. The next day we were told she had a terrible accident. She had tried to fix soup for herself because both her parents were at work. As she climbed up on the counter to get a bowl, the sash of her dress caught fire. We had not been instructed to stop, drop, and roll. The fire worked its way up her back as she went running out into the street screaming for help. She was burned severely. Judy was one of my best friends, and I missed her terribly. When I did get to see her, the back of her arms and legs and her whole back was scarred. I wonder today whatever happened to her. The scars surely made her life difficult. Wherever you are, Judy, I hope you are okay.

Wheel going around and around, clicking, spinning, driving
me further into life, away from, toward. Where have I

> *begun, where have I been, where am I going? I just keep*
> *pedaling, around and around … I saw what I saw, I see*
> *what I see, I will see what there is to see. Oh, wheel going*
> *around and around, clicking, spinning, driving me further,*
> *further, further … When I stop, nobody knows; where I*
> *stop I know not either. I just am, I just am, I … just … am.*
> *I … am … I am … I … I … I … am … am … am …*

Fifth grade was the beginning of my worse years. I had both my appendix and my tonsils out in one year. Being in the hospital twice—and they kept you in a long time in those days—there was something about being taken care of by doctors and nurses that made me want to call out to them, "Can you help me? Can you *please* help me?" I did not know what I needed help with; I just needed something to help me feel better. To make things worse, I had a teacher who talked about you to the other students, for whatever reason, when you were out sick. This was definitely the year that the shame planted in me took root. When I was in school, I stared out the window constantly, so much so that the teacher sent notes home to my parents. I wondered what she expected them to do.

One student, John Boward, was always catching head colds. It made my eyes water to hear him read aloud and I would not even look over at him for fear the snot was dripping onto the page. I would think to myself, *Couldn't someone please get a wrench and fix his spigot?* Of course, his mother kept him home a lot. The teacher made it sound like he was a hopeless hypochondriac, which of course he wasn't. He just got sick more than most. I don't know what she said about me in my absence. It probably doesn't matter.

I was glad to get to sixth grade. Miss Kegris gave me reason to believe in myself, like I was a capable learner and a whole person. I remember putting my hand up to give the meaning of the word "mutiny," and I was praised for this. Also, this was my first year in the school choir. I remember struggling because even the simplest lyrics were difficult for me to learn. I knew the music, and I knew what the words were, but I could not seem to put them together very successfully. This discouraged me. Was I somehow different from the other kids? I could not understand.

Seventh grade at Edison Junior High School was very different from little ole all-white Melrose Elementary, not only that it was a much bigger school and with more rules. We moved from room to room for the different class periods. I felt so lost those first few months. I hung together with my friend Susan from Melrose and two other friends, Jeanie and Joanne. We were birds of a feather. We loved pajama parties and slang books. In case you've not heard of a slang book, it is simply a tablet with a student's name on every page, and it would be passed around for people to put their distorted opinions down about each person. Kids could be cruel.

We never had detention at Melrose either. But at Edison, sometimes you were made to stay after school if you had acted out or talked during class. And kids were paddled there too! I will never forget Mr. Kunkle's math class in eighth grade. My friend Susan sat in front of me, and at one point she pretended to swallow the white pearl button off her sweater. I let out a gasp and soon found myself waiting in the hall—was I going to be paddled? I almost wet my pants. But all I got was a scolding, along with missing part of a lesson.

I could not explain why moving in lines from class to class was so disconcerting for me. Even though it was only a matter of following the person in front of me, I felt lost and bewildered. Where was I, what was I doing, and who were all these strange people? Gym class was smelly with sweat, and we had to take showers together. There were only two girls to a stall, but I did not care for even that much exposure. Fortunately, my good friend Susan was my shower partner. Still, there were a lot of boobs flying around the room. We all compared bra sizes a good bit. Susan's and mine seemed to be among the smallest. The shiny, wet bodies of the black girls were beautiful, but they were a great deal more verbal, and they scared me some.

My seventh-grade home room teacher, Mrs. Hummer, was a sweet older woman. She could be very reassuring, and I needed that. I remember being told our class was one of the two with higher IQs. I did not feel that intelligent. Then one day Mr. Dickey, who taught history in a classroom on the lower level, challenged us to learn all fifty counties in Pennsylvania. He was quite a character. I aced the test. Maybe I was a little bright. Mr. Dickey was more of a standup comedian than a teacher, and the fifty-minute class went by too fast. It was one place I felt invitingly comfortable, if not a little let down by how little we actually learned there.

I enjoyed gym class since I was hyperactive. I just did not enjoy what it did to me. Mrs. Study insisted our white cotton uniforms be fresh and clean.

We would soak our white canvas sneakers in shoe polish. Our uniform, sneakers, towel, soap, fresh underwear—everything was stuffed into a small, hard cosmetic case. Susan and I toted them with a dozen or so heavy books ten blocks to school in the morning and back home in the afternoon. It was a real test of strength, one that left me feeling broken at the end of the day. It took a couple of days to recover from gym day, only to repeat the whole process again at the end of the week. Life felt literally impossible to me, but I could not explain what I was feeling to anyone. It was misery—pure, simple *misery*.

There were some really loud and wild gangs at Edison. One day a group of kids found the head to a doll on the school grounds. Someone covered it with red lipstick, and a number of kids were kicking it around, making a sport of it. One young lady—I guess you could call her a lady—declared it the head of her unborn baby. It was disgusting. Later Mr. Study, the boys' gym teacher, and a number of other teachers were trying to establish who was involved in this little illicit sport. My friends pointed to me, even though I had just been an observer. I was never punished, but let me tell you, I stayed away from any large, rambunctious groups after that.

I dreaded the thought of even getting detention. I was once sent to detention with our whole geography class but managed to put it completely out of my lame head. I could not explain forgetting such a thing. I went straight home after school with not a single thought about it. My mother had to talk to the assistant principal the next day to get me out of trouble. Not by far would this be the last time my mother would come to my rescue. She would have made a good lawyer.

I had Mr. McLamb for English. He was my first black and male teacher, and I was sure he had it in for me. I got a warning card mid-semester. For the first time I was going to get a D on my report card. Again, my mother became involved in my pathetic life by coming to school to talk to him. Apparently she told him how afraid I was of him. He came to me and explained, "I like you just fine, Sylvia." For our next assignment we were to write a diary for Longfellow's epic poem, "Evangeline." I put myself in that boat, floating down the St. Lawrence River. And I put my heart—her heart—on paper, placing it between the carefully designed front and back covers with a piece of yellow yarn tying it all together. Well, that was all it took. From then on in I got an A+ in his class. And I fell head over heels into pleasing this kind black gentleman.

When I was twelve, Mother encouraged me to sign up for a Red Cross course in home nursing. She felt since I was to be a nurse this would be a good experience. We learned how to take temperatures and to give bed baths. They instructed us on the five ways disease is spread: flies, fingers, feces, faces, and food. And when we were done, we were officially qualified to become candy stripers. I began going to the county nursing home. Mostly I emptied bedpans, gave a few baths, and fed people, crying my whole way home. Mother said to me, "Sylvia, if it makes you so sad why do you go there?" My tearful reply was, "Well, someone has to cheer them up." Nothing felt cheerful behind my smiles. In a way *it* cheered me. Once I took a double-hearted yellow rose. I must have shown the rose to a hundred people that day. Indeed it did lift my heart. There were days when I did not want to get out of bed. I pushed myself to move, and I pretended I was on a stage. I had to act my part. It was here, too, that I learned how polio could rampage a person's life.

One of the guests at the county home was a relatively young black woman by the name of Ruthie Peterson. She had been in a wheelchair since contracting polio at the age of nine, but there was not a note of bitterness in this dear woman; she compensated for her confinement by being the center of social life at the home. Everybody loved Ruthie. Her face lit up many a time as her lilting voice sang glorious hymns, thus breaking through the clouds around and above me and bringing a bit of sunshine to all who were in her presence.

> *Wheel going around and around, clicking, spinning, driving*
> *me further into life, away from, toward. Where have I*
> *begun, where have I been, where am I going? I just keep*
> *pedaling, around and around ... I saw what I saw, I see*
> *what I see, I will see what there is to see. Oh, wheel going*
> *around and around, clicking, spinning, driving me further,*
> *further, further ... When I stop, nobody knows; where I*
> *stop I know not either. I just am, I just am, I ... just ... am.*
> *I ... am ... I am ... I ... I ... I ... am ... am ... am ...*

Up to this point, our family had still been residing in the city. After Edison, I went to John Harris High School in the city for only a month. High school was just another confusing place to me. Our homeroom teacher read to us from John Bunyan's *Pilgrim's Progress* each morning before sending us into the day. For some reason, this story stayed in my mind and revisited me *down the road*. The story instilled a sense of hope in me, and I needed this. Then it happened—someone threw another wrench into the works. We moved to the suburbs. I wanted to stay with my friends in the city schools, but I had to spend my last three years of public school among strangers. It felt like such a curse.

Susquehanna Township Senior High School had the usual cliques, none of which I seemed to fit. I had been singing in choirs since sixth grade, so I gravitated to their choir. The director, Miss Lindemuth, was another sort of tall, lanky woman. I still could barely fit the notes with the lyrics without great confusion. I sensed something was wrong with my head, but I had no idea what it was.

Gym, again, was a problem. Like a gym teacher does, Mrs. Florry made us run a lot. If we were not running around the tennis courts, we were running around the gym. I would have the class on a Tuesday, and it would take until Friday for the spasms in my face, and now chest pain, to subside, only to have to run again. My life was an endless feeling of recovering and then having to repeat the offending behavior and recover again. I became more and more hyperactive. While waiting for a bus downtown, I recall my brother asking me, "Sylvia, do you ever hold still?" But when I was hurting, oftentimes the only thing that helped was pumping an endless stream of adrenalin to get on top of the feelings, whatever they were. I was clueless as to the nature of this insanity in my life.

By high school, I was already dead. Nothing mattered much to me by then, and not my social life especially. Physical activity was important to me. I had to stay strong because I felt like I was in a race for my life. I had to win. But where was I going and why? It is hard for me to even look at these years without bringing up some old, painful memories. But now I have to look at a part of my life that haunted me and taunted me, almost sending me into oblivion. Here goes: nursing.

Nurse Nancy

I was accepted into a local nursing school out of high school. No one asked me if this is what I wanted. I had been labeled, "the nurse", since I was five years old for the simple reason I played intently with a little plastic doctor's kit: stethoscope, reflex hammer, thermometer, and wristwatch. Father referred to me lovingly as "Nurse Nancy" after a character in one of my children's Golden Books. I guess I just looked the part. I knew very little of what I was getting myself into. Oh, I had cared plenty for sick folk, but I never really looked at medicine as a profession. I just gravitated into it. The rigors of nursing, especially as the work dogs we were as students in the '60s, was getting to be way more than I could handle. On weekends in the hospital it was not unusual to be given eight, ten, or even twelve patients to care for. On top of the usual head and face spasms accompanied by strange, annoying chest pain, I would leave work in the evening with my legs aching like crazy. Sore legs and feet are a given in nursing.

One Sunday I came back to school from a weekend at home, bringing my bicycle. I began riding whenever I got a chance. After this I no longer had the leg and foot pain, only the usual agony from all the lifting and arm work. I often felt I was in more pain than my sickest patients. I was a basket case inside. But I kept it all bottled up inside me, trying hard not to show what I felt. I was literally dying emotionally inside, and I could tell no one.

Polyclinic Hospital School of Nursing was a three-year diploma school, of which I completed only two years. The instructors, in my eyes, were teachers from hell. They taught by scare tactics. "If you don't do [this] then [that] will happen." Geesh, didn't I have enough fear in my life already? By then I had been secretly depressed for eight years. This strange breed, nurse instructors, seemed more like a nasty brood of spinsters. The older sister to one of my brother's friends was among them. When Barbara walked into a room, it grew instantly chilly. It is a wonder ice did not form on the windows. I don't think I wanted to be like any of them. I had thought I wanted to be a psychiatric nurse, but a three-month rotation at our local Harrisburg State Hospital cured me of that false hope. In the back of my mind I think I wanted mostly to figure out my own thinking.

Grace, one of the beauticians who did Mother's hair, had a mother in one of the back wards of the hospital. There were few drugs to help with mental illness in the '60s, so these people were simply kept like beasts, farmed into back wards. It was at this time I knew I was as screwed up in my head as some of the patients I was working with as a student. One was just a kid in what they called the "receiving area" for whom I worked out "the perfect treatment plan"—like I knew it all, do you think? When I shared my plan in class, it got shot out of the air like a clay pigeon. I was stricken. I quit. I mean I really quit and was out of the nurses' dormitory the next day, leaving a not-so-likeable roommate in the tailwind. The irony was, my first roommate there, Barbara, and I wrote the new alma mater for the school to the tune of, "Let There Be Music." Both of us quit shortly afterward.

Alma Mater for Polyclinic Hospital School of Nursing
[1968, to the tune of "Let There Be Music"]
Where there is pain and suf'ering in the world,
There be our souls' domain;
Ev-ery prayer within our hearts is for the good of man.
May we our skill and knowledge yield to a cause,
Worthy of humble praise.
May we as nurses of God's land yield forth our rev'rent hands.
The Polyclinic nurses strive to reach those goals so high,
that life's most trying challenges will all be overcome.
There's a spirit in our voices and faith that leads us on,
To follow in the steps of those whose wisdom made us strong.
May we with the healing hand of God,
Sustain the gift of life.

After two years in this place that put such a great physical and emotional demand on me, about all I was left with was a sense of being able to make people *feel better*. I could not necessarily make them feel better physically but emotionally. I would give a super back rub, and I knew the words to soothe them. That is probably why I hung on as long as I did at the school. However, when it came to the actual nursing, I somehow could not do it. One example was when I was on the operating room rotation.

I had a ninety-six-year-old man who had a supra-pubic prostatectomy for a case study. In other words, they took his prostate gland out by an incision through the abdomen. I was to stay with him through his surgery and recovery, had that been possible. I was faced with the equivalent of him

40

urinating through a drain in the incision. I must have changed his dressing a hundred times in eight hours, maybe more. Now mind you, the supply room was only across the hall and up two doors. To have been really *practical*, I would have stocked a rolling supply cart with cartons of dressings. Instead, I proceeded to run back and forth, back and forth … more dressings, more tape, more dressings, more tape … Maybe I am imagining things, but I swore that supply room was getting further and further from the man's hospital bed. It didn't matter anyway; he died that night. I had never in my life felt so inadequate.

DIVE FOR SAFETY

I did not realize how much tension had so thoroughly worked its way into my body and psyche over those two years that I call hell now. In the middle of my first night home, I lay sleepless, wondering what was to become of me. I went out to the living room and put on one of my father's records. As Handel's "He Shall Feed His Flocks" played quietly, I lay on the floor sobbing my heart out. I felt the tension drain from my body. When it was over, I was even more certain nursing was *not* for me—for a time, that is. I knew nothing of where I was going. At this point I didn't care.

Many of my high school classmates were married. Even a number of former nursing classmates were married too. I had no boyfriends; they seemed off my radar. I had had a couple over the years, but they only left me feeling more dispassionate. In high school my cousin Stanley, who was a missionary in South America, hooked me up with a friend of his named Alphonso from Bogotá, Columbia. This man slobbered all over me. It took me eight years to convince him I was not going to marry him and move to South America with him. Another young guy, Richard, followed me around for a while in high school. I could not explain my disinterest in lovers or sex. I guess the chemistry was just not there. I would come to understand it many years later. I even considered that maybe I was gay, but I liked men too much.

Following nursing school, I got another chance for higher education, wherever it was to lead. We had had two community college instructors in nursing school for English Composition I and II. One of them, Mr. Elmy, was just the sweetest little guy who was impressed by my writing.

I felt some promise in becoming a writer, although I had no idea what I would write about. As much as I loved reading over the years, I never had the concentration to actually read and get much out of it. Hell, I could not even read a newspaper; the news upset me too much inside—even the good news. Over the years I heard Mother and Father discuss and write editorials. But it always, again, confused me. Why was I always strapped for clear thoughts?

How could I write if I had no real voice or opinion? All I really knew was my own sense of stupidity. I was simple minded and going nowhere. It was no wonder I had quit in my senior year of nursing school. Senior students were on the hospital departments at night, often alone in making life-or-death decisions. How was I to do this if I could not make a single decision for myself? Up to this point I had always been told what to do, where to do it, and how. I had no reason to think for myself.

> *Wheel going around and around, clicking, spinning, driving*
> *me further into life, away from, toward. Where have I*
> *begun, where have I been, where am I going? I just keep*
> *pedaling, around and around ... I saw what I saw, I see*
> *what I see, I will see what there is to see. Oh, wheel going*
> *around and around, clicking, spinning, driving me further,*
> *further, further ... When I stop, nobody knows; where I*
> *stop I know not either. I just am, I just am, I ... just ... am.*
> *I ... am ... I am ... I ... I ... I ... am ... am ... am ...*

Mother, again, made the appointment for me to see an intake counselor at the community college. I slid into communication and the arts and did royally. I joined the college newspaper, served as recording secretary in student government, worked in the activities office, and even chaired the activities committee for a summer. One of the older students, Mrs. Tamanini, a middle-aged mother of four, did a weekly column with me called, "The Bridge Builder." We decided we would interview faculty, especially the newer members, and share it with the rest of the campus. This was exciting, and I got to show some of my colors. The faculty seemed to open up to us easily. I was at the top of my game, but there was still a feeling something was wrong with me.

I spent too much time in the distribution department, taking the papers to each department, running across campus and up and down stairs. By the time I was done, I was in so much pain that it was all I could do to study. Any sane person would have understood, "I just cannot do these things." But I understood so little of what I was feeling—where it came from, why ... why ... why? I don't know how I had a 3.4 GPA. It must have been osmosis.

I had a couple of guys trailing behind me. I even went out more than once with a fellow named Terry, who I could just barely stand. In my second year, the mother of our newspaper editor, Jim, committed suicide. I could see the grief etched in the face of this pleasant young man. He came to me, reached out to me, and I turned him away like a cold-hearted bitch. I felt bad about it at the time, but something inside held me back. Years later I would thoroughly understand why our relationship would have been bad—really bad.

I graduated in 1970 with my name in *Who's Who of American Junior Colleges* and a leadership award. But none of this spoke for who I really was inside. I was depressed, broken, and sick, sick, sick ... I gravitated to a four-year college, but I got so depressed by the end of the first semester that I quit—again. Again? Damn!

I got a job as a nurse technician, the equivalent of a practical nurse, because of my two years of nurse's training. I even signed up and began nursing school again at the very college from which I had just graduated. My life seemed like an endless cycle of stops and starts and stops and starts. I would try and try again. What on earth was wrong with me? Soon I was about to find out a lot about myself—things I did not want to know. And I was about to make some of the worst decisions a person could make.

For someone with severe chest pain from lifting, it made no sense at all to be working as a nurse and trying to study at the same time. I had no ability to stop. What was it Sir Isaac Newton said—"An object in motion tends to stay in motion, unless acted upon by an equal and opposing force"? Well, I was about to go into overdrive, with no brakes on my *car*.

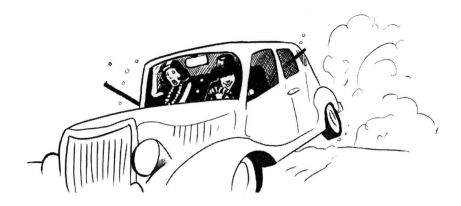

Chapter 2

I've Got a Brand-New Pair of Roller Skates, You've Got a Brand-New Key

*Wheel going around and around, clicking, spinning, driving
me further into life, away from, toward. Where have I
begun, where have I been, where am I going? I just keep
pedaling, around and around … I saw what I saw, I see
what I see, I will see what there is to see. Oh, wheel going
around and around, clicking, spinning, driving me further,
further, further … When I stop, nobody knows; where I
stop I know not either. I just am, I just am, I … just … am.
I … am … I am … I … I … I … am … am … am …*

Wheels—roller skates, bicycles, and automobiles—dominated my
life. Derry Street, right out in front of our building, was the site of
accident after accident. People would get hit by cars. One day a woman with
a chocolate milkshake in her hand was sent flying into the air, milkshake
all over the offending vehicle, her, and the street. Our street was the main
thoroughfare for ambulances and fire engines. Just up the street, outside
Goodyear's Pharmacy, was the intersection of three different streets,

regulated by a traffic signal. The city bus line stopped on the corner just across the street.

My first memory of being in a car was in the old family Studebaker. It had stalled downtown and Father could not get it started. Cars were not as efficient in the late 1940s and '50s. As a small child, I remember sitting on the grey woolen front seat one winter wishing we could get home and get warm. We had a family car for all of the years I recall. One of my favorites was an aquamarine-colored Nash Rambler with the spare tire encased and mounted on the rear. Nor did we have seatbelts in those days. I almost lost an eye to testify to this truth.

As was often the case, I was out in one of the business cars with Jim, the delivery boy, when we came to a sudden stop. I was in the back, and there was a metal coil protruding from the back of the front seat. It just missed my right eye, but I had a pretty nasty cut at the inner corner of my eye. Yes, sudden stops and fender benders were almost a norm for us. Those "boys" were like our baby sitters when we were still toddlers. For many years we children got to go on the rounds. In other words, we would accompany Mother or Father on a trip south to Gettysburg, Hanover, and Lancaster, or north to Lewisberry, Sunbury, and Shamokin to service the many dealerships with posters advertising Fine Art Photo and Kodak film and in search of lost orders. These were pictures that ended up in the wrong hands or, worse yet, in no hands. This could be a nightmare for my parents. However, the personnel at the stores were friendly. While Mother or Father were going through box after box of orders, we got to peruse the stores, sampling colognes, sipping an occasional soda, or with soft wads of Double Bubble in our mouths.

Wheels definitely made life interesting. As teenagers the delivery boys left us off at the Capitol, and we got to run the route by foot and take photo orders in a brown satchel to the snack bars in various government buildings. One of a number of blind proprietors, Gus Walkhouse, knew me just by the time of day and my footsteps. I remember getting off the elevator on the fourteenth floor and he was standing at the entrance to the snack bar. He greeted me with, "Hi, Sylvia, any photos for us today?"

At the end of our run through four different buildings, up and down elevators or staircases, we would stand in front of Murphy's Five and Dime Store waiting for the bus to take us home. Downtown Harrisburg, especially around Christmas or Easter, was lit up and decorated. Pomeroy's on the corner of Fourth and Market Streets had display windows filled with moving characters and colorful props. Family and children crowded around to feast their eyes on the elves and Santa. Yes, we got around real well, but as my teenage years dwindled and adolescence crept in, I began using wheels more for escape than for the fun.

Escape? Escape from what? For anyone to look at me, like my brother's friends who seemed to enjoy feasting their eyes on me, I was normal. I felt "fat," like a lot of Barbie-doll generation girls felt as a rule. But I did not have an eating disorder. I ate well—I had to, to sustain my level of activity. I moved from the time I awoke in the morning until I hit the sack at night. But by the age of sixteen, I was increasingly unable to sleep at night. My brain felt like it was on hyper-alert, like if I closed my eyes something horrible was going to happen to me. I recall one particularly difficult night.

It was summer, and I was at my aunt's house in Harrisburg. I had been romping in the yard that evening, turning summersaults and cartwheels, one after the other. That night I lay in their back bedroom staring out the overhead window at the starry sky. I was thinking how clear the sky was, and the full moon lit my room. At the same time I was also thinking, *What am I feeling? What is it in me that can make me so happy and so miserable at the same time? Why does my head feel like it will split, and why do I have chest pain like I am going to have a heart attack? What is it in me that wants to live and to die, both at once?* I lay there all night with my eyes wide open, laughing and crying. I had long since stopped saying, "I hurt." No one took me seriously anyway. This is when my *wheels* started to turn out of control.

One weekend after a second and failed semester at Millersville University, I had been at my grandparents' house. I got there in one of my father's old delivery cars, a little red Renault. And I had a full tank of gas. It was the afternoon of a beautiful day, and the rolling hills of Cumberland County enticed me to keep driving and driving. I had no destination—I just drove and drove and drove … The sun went down, and I still drove. I was lost and found in a little car destined to go nowhere and everywhere. I was twenty-three years old, and I wanted to show Mother and Father I could make a difference.

By this time Father had partly retired from the business. They still had a mail-order business in the basement of our home in the suburbs. If

I had wanted to, I could have become more involved with this. But there was no glamour, nothing enticing me to get involved. There was always something I could do to help, but I wanted more than anything just to get away from Mother. She had a way about her that sent people scurrying away when they saw her coming. She had an agenda, and everyone knew it. The only way I knew to get away was to get a job and move to the other side of the Susquehanna River. Surely that would cut the infernal umbilical cord between us.

I had tunnel vision when it came to finding work. Nursing was all I knew, so I got a job on that side of the river too—at the hospital. At the same time, I signed up for the nursing course at the community college. And I found a young woman named Judy who wanted someone to share her apartment. She had a sweet six-year-old daughter named Kendra. It seemed ideal, so I moved in.

Our apartment was in a huge complex of apartments. I didn't know people could hear so much in a place like that. They could. So there I was, going to school in the daytime and working evenings at the hospital. Surely now I would learn to think for myself and find some badly needed autonomy, although I must admit I was clueless about the latter. My mother was respected and listened to by so many, and I felt I had so much of her in me. But there was a part of me also that wanted nothing to do with her. Father had always been the "silent partner" in our home, and he was the part of me I wanted to get to know better.

> Wheel going around and around, clicking, spinning, driving
> me further into life, away from, toward. Where have I
> begun, where have I been, where am I going? I just keep
> pedaling, around and around ... I saw what I saw, I see
> what I see, I will see what there is to see. Oh, wheel going
> around and around, clicking, spinning, driving me further,
> further, further ... When I stop, nobody knows; where I
> stop I know not either. I just am, I just am, I ... just ... am.
> I ... am ... I am ... I ... I ... I ... am ... am ... am ...

This living arrangement was new to me, but I honestly felt it just might work. And so it began—the coming and going, coming and going, coming and going. I would work ten days straight at the hospital, and then they would call me on my day off to come in to work. This is what happened on that day I found myself maneuvering the hills of Cumberland County. I think I was looking for a place to land. A coworker had befriended me, but when her boyfriend took an interest in me, she literally came at me, fisticuffs, like a bat out of hell. I was doubly—no, triply—no, quadruple vexed and crushed.

My work at the hospital involved not only lifting and turning heavy patients but also running room-to-room counting the drops of intravenous feedings. No, there were no handy little machines to do this, like there are today. On one particularly busy evening, I had run so far, and on hard concrete floors, that I snapped a bone in my left foot. I had it x-rayed, but there are so many bones in the foot all they could tell me was it was a "stress fracture" and nothing could be done about it. So, I just limped my way through the rest of the eight-hour shift.

Most evenings I was to do treatments on two different halls of the fourth floor, a medical department. The halls intersected as the work crucified me. The ache in me was so deep and complete—I was working in a Catholic hospital; surely the nuns knew what they were doing to me. I did not hear about or see that other nurses were feeling my agony. Were they? I thought, *Surely I am no different than them, so I may as well just do my work and suck up these feelings!*

I was doing the work of an unlicensed practical nurse, but I don't think I was ever really very practical at all. I would run to one patient room to do a treatment, only to realize I was missing an essential supply, or instrument pack. Why was I so reckless and at a loss for coordination? Needless to say, this doubled or tripled my work. Any sane person would have known just to get out. But mind you, I *was ... not ... sane*. Many a night I would spin my wheels at work, tears dripping from my cheeks the whole way home. I cried through the night, and even if I slept at all, in the morning I felt a heavy ache in my chest. I had grown way too familiar with the clouds of depression lingering over my head. Yes, even on sunny days there were *insufferable* clouds! What was wrong with me? Why all the sadness?

After a month of trying to work and go to school at the same time, I must have started to look pretty haggard. Dear Mother, and her mothering instincts, as usual honed in and had me see the good Dr. Bennet, who prescribed a heavy sleeping pill. By this time my nights and days were starting to run together. The pills did nothing to help me sleep. At one point I recall not sleeping for three weeks straight. I didn't know someone could stay awake that long. I thrashed around in bed all night or stood by the window sobbing, looking obliviously into the night. This was when a whole new chapter in my life was about to unfold. I was about to learn a lesson I did not expect. This is when I crash landed ... on *Mars*.

THE ANTICS OF *BONNIE AND CLYDE*

It was about 8:00 p.m. on an October evening. I was at work, and I noticed Mrs. McQueen, the woman at the end of the hall, still had a visitor in her room. Visiting hours were over, so I stepped in to remind them. The bed light was on over her head, and in front of her stood a young man with sandy brown hair and blue eyes that sparkled. He had a look of desperation mixed with mischief written on his slightly unshaven face. We may have exchanged formalities; I barely recall. His name was Sam. But feeling like a wild cat with parched lips being drawn to a deep oasis, I walked out of there with an address on a piece of paper in my pocket. I was to pick him up after work.

I was not surprised at his loneliness. What man living with his mother, who was in the hospital, wouldn't be lonely? Something happened to me that evening. He sat sipping brews and me margaritas at a local pub. From the jukebox somewhere Melanie was belting out her colorful lyrics, "I have a brand-new pair of roller skates, you have a brand-new key ... I think that we should get together 'nd try them out and see ..."

I could not explain my inability to resist this man's advances. I was being drawn into a bottomless chasm. In fact, I was drowning, and I didn't care. I had never been that close—that intimate—with a man. This man was not just any man. I wanted him more than I could recall ever wanting anything in my life. Surely he was God's gift to me. Would he rescue me from myself? I needed someone to take me away from everything, everyone—take me someplace, everyplace, and no place, all at once. And he did too. Nothing mattered but the passion I saw and felt from those hazel blue eyes.

Over drinks, he seemed to be mumbling, fumbling for words. He was trying to tell me something. I didn't care what deep, dark secrets he had. All I cared about was the feel of his skin next to mine, him entering me in a way no man had ever done. Suddenly that cat by the oasis no longer had parched lips, and there was no turning back. Each beat of my heart brought me closer to his. I was a prisoner of the heart, and it felt *so good*. Soon there would be no way to turn back, but I did not care in the least. My captor could do anything—take me anywhere—and it would be okay.

My father's little red Renault carried us all over town, up and down hills through, again, Cumberland County. It seemed to not matter where we were going. All that mattered was the privacy. Sam seemed frightened, like he would be trapped if we stopped. I sensed talk was the enemy. In a way it felt like I was becoming the rescuer. Instead of the usual love duo where the lad rescues the maiden, this maiden was rescuing her lad. (What is wrong with this picture?) It did not matter. Someone had lit my fire, and after just one evening together, I committed myself—correction, I *commuted* myself—to something I could not take back. Suddenly the quiet misery in me that had kept me suffering year after year dissolved. The job, the classes to get my RN ("Registered Nut" to my mind), and proving myself to my parents meant nothing. I had the "roller skates"; he had the "key." The journey had just begun.

I awoke the next morning, not surprisingly, with my first hangover. Up until that night neither had I been intimate with a man, nor had I drank margaritas as if I were emptying the river basin. (I liked them.) I found out, too, that the Susquehanna River was not wide enough nor deep enough to separate Mother from my life. She called at 7:30 a.m. It was a Saturday morning and my day off!

"Sylvia, I need you to come home and help us with zip codes in the basement." My mother, the business woman, was still the *busyness* woman and my boss.

"No, Mother, this is my day off. I haven't slept." I did not tell her I had been awake for three weeks. "I'm tired, I don't feel well, and I have a new friend I must see."

She never could hear the word no. Never. At this point, I think I just totally numbed myself. I snapped, slamming the phone back onto the receiver. I was so frightened inside, needing to rescue myself from this ominous beast I sensed rising from deep inside. What was I feeling? What was I doing? In my mind I put that woman, my mother, on the do not call list. I immediately called Sam, needing to know he was there for me. But instead of a sympathetic ear on the other end of the phone, I was met with the voice of desperation.

"Sylvia, I have to leave town."

"Why, Sam? Where are you going? Why do you have to leave? We just met. Please don't leave. Please ..."

I recalled during one of our intimate moments the night before, he had mentioned that he had an older brother, Clarence, who was in prison. Any sane person would have pursued a line of questioning here. Just what kind of family *was* he coming from? I knew he and his mother were both heavy smokers—Lucky Strikes—and I knew he liked Southern brew—Busch Beer in particular. He had spoken to me of Florida like it was the next state down and as if he may have had acquaintances there.

"I just have to go, Sylvia." I think he spoke my name personally, maybe not. It didn't matter.

"Sam, if you are going I am going too ... We'll take *my* car."

As a result of three weeks of insomnia, I had all my Christmas shopping done. That day I wrapped eight gifts, got all my affairs in line, and visited Sister Jonathan, director of nursing at the hospital, to tell her I needed to take a leave. I had only been working there for nine months, but I was burned out. My nerves were raw, and I wanted to explode. Instead I was imploding. On top of it all, Sam had sparked a whole new set of feelings. Had I a confidant and had he or she asked, I don't think I could have found the words to put it all together. "What's going on, Sylvia?" But there wasn't anyone asking. It was just me, God, and Sam ... I somehow persuaded him to wait until evening.

"Then you, me, and our little red Renault will be 'King of the Road.' Destination: Florida."

Had he not hung up so quickly, I would have added, "Or anyplace else your frightened heart and male body desires we should go. I don't care where we are going or what you have done, we'll go together."

By evening I had written notes to my family about what to do with my little bit of furnishings and personal belongings in the apartment. In my mind, the decision I had just made to run away with a young man whom I barely knew and with a shady past made all the sense in the world. It made sense because so much of what I was feeling in my body—spasms in my face and neck accompanied by severe chest pain and burning—made absolutely no sense. To my sleep-deprived mind, this new plan made sense. I would tell no one, especially my mother, for fear she as always would try to censor my thoughts. Nope, this was *my* decision, and I wanted everybody else out of my head and out of my way!

Darkness had, by now, become like an old friend, but not the kind of friend one would want to invite over for dinner with the folks. Nor was my new companion someone I wanted Mom and Dad to meet. His language was rough, and he smoked; those two things alone were unacceptable in any friend, but in a man friend, especially, they would be taboo. Besides, I had done the unthinkable; I had had sex out of wedlock! Most twenty-three-year-olds would not have given their parents much credence, but mind you, Mother and Father saw me still as their canary in the church choir loft. I could not sing a sour note. I was their cherub, and I knew they would not approve of this restless, unkempt young man.

Mind you, also, up to this point I was still unable to make decisions for myself, but no one had ever asked exactly why this was. I quite honestly felt deep down there was something wrong with me, but I was clueless as to what. Had anyone asked me directly, I would probably have told them, "Sylvia is not right in the head." I had full-blown head spasms and chest pain—constant chest pain—from working. I was in so much pain I could barely put two and two together and get four. I knew the answers to a lot of questions. I just did not know how I got them. Yes, there were definitely some screws loose somewhere.

By 4:00 p.m. I was ready. My anticipation peaked, I sat waiting at the top of the musky-smelling, stagnant apartment stairwell. The *man*—a man unlike any I had known before him—would be at my door soon. I don't know why he would not let me pick him up. Today I would have guessed someone must be hot on this man's trail. But at the time nothing mattered except my one-track-mind decision to follow him to the end of the earth.

There I was, perched like a bird on the top step of the apartment vestibule, waiting on her flock to migrate south. It had grown dark outside. Behind me in the apartment lay a carefully planned-out note that was to account for just about everything I owned—my parents' old bedroom set, a desk and chair, an old dining room table I had antiqued with two old chairs, and most sacred, a collection of various books, few of which I had been able to read because I simply needed the time and the peace of mind. The Christmas gifts for my family were wrapped and stacked neatly in the closet. My life was in a nutshell, and I was ready for whatever God had in store for me. Whatever it was, it had to be better than those weeks—no, years—of torment I was leaving behind.

As I waited, I ran up and down that musty-smelling, closed stairwell, hoping, wishing he would get there. I kept thinking, *Maybe he changed his mind and went without me.* After all, I had only known him less than forty-eight hours. Why should he even care about me? Did he feel the surging, ebbing passion I felt? If he didn't, what reason would he have to come for me? Surely I would be extra baggage, a ball and chain around his ankle. Just then, I heard the heavy door open below. His deep voice echoed up, "Sylvia, are you there?" I grabbed the small backpack from beside me, supposedly containing everything I would need for my journey, just the basics. Our departure had to be quick and quiet. And there would be no turning back.

This pristine point of departure was like diving on a hot, humid day into the depths of a cool mountain stream, cleansing myself of all the negativity and feelings of low self-worth. Nothing would ever be the same. Life would never be the same because I had lost the innocence of yesterday in exchange for the promise of who I was becoming. And this was what made the journey so valuable. I was just beginning to open the treasure chest of my own being, of a subconscious so full of promise. This was *both a beginning and an ending, thus altering all time.* It was an *affirmation of rebirth, which seemed to go back but really went forward. It undid the past in the present, thus releasing the future.*[iii] My destiny was unlocked. A waiting world had its arms out to receive me, and yet I felt I was falling, falling, falling … and it took my breath away.

In spite of the apprehension, somehow, at this point I was sure of what I was doing and that it was the answer to my desperation. And I was sure *we* would do just fine *down the road*—wherever that was. Sam insisted on driving. I let him. He seemed edgy and determined to evade something. Looking back, he just may have told me about the reality that was about to slap me in the face: he was a felon, a car thief, and the police wanted him. He may have told me this. I very well may have been listening—yes, I probably was. In fact, this kind of rebellious, sociopath personality was probably what attracted me to him. By being the middle child for so many years, I had been extremely compliant but at the same time the least capable of getting what I wanted. I was a parent pleaser and a sibling peacemaker. These things are only clear to me today after almost forty years of retrospection. A lot of denial still lay ahead at this point in my story. Go ahead, shake your head and go, "Tsk, tsk"—I deserve it.

It was dark as we drove down Route 15 South. I was exhausted, wound too tightly, and about to break like an old clock. The further down the road we got, the more I sensed a coil slowly unfurling inside of me, freeing me of months of pain, exhaustion, and yes, more constant than anything, the depression. By this time in my life, depression was my most intimate friend. I did not ask for the relationship; I inherited it. We drove into the cool, darkening night, just barely able to see the fall foliage on both sides of the road. He took command of the wheel like an experienced driver, me sitting peacefully beside him and with the clean scent of his Aramis mesmerizing my tormented mind. It was then I began to feel something I had not known up until leaving that barren apartment behind and any thoughts of my overbearing mother—that tight coil in my gut, slowly, slowly unfurling, relaxing.

I was a dove in the presence of a hawk, but he was tender and caring toward me. I had no concern about my welfare. At that pristine point of departure, Sam was my newfound protector. Soon the agony and extreme exhaustion would be replaced by a sense of purpose. He asked me, "Do you believe two people can live on love alone?" After a pause he finished, "I do."

I responded quietly a minute later, "Yes, Sam, I believe it."

I was feeling a surge of newfound happiness, a kind of energy to replace what had drained almost totally from my being. I was in what felt like love—the deepest, most profound state of *love*. I must say here, however, there was one other factor that motivated us into this kind of insane, wanton journey. We drank. I mean we really drank—hard. We put away more beer and mixed drinks in those few days together than I knew any two human beings could consume. We never had alcohol in our home growing up. Now every swallow of the pungent liquid left me feeling powerful, able to handle anything. A false sense of well being and near total lack of inhibition left me unable to choose wisely.

Had I not been drinking with Sam—well, number one, he probably would not have wanted anything to do with me. And number two, I also would have dropped him like a hot potato. I had never before defied Mother's control, nor had I challenged my father's subservience toward her. Taking life into my own hands was a new feeling. I correct myself here: I placed my life recklessly into the hands of this *Don Quixote*.

I had a checkbook but only about $150 in the account. This helped fill the gas tank and get us to his aunt and uncle's house in Columbia, North Carolina. Sam seemed comfortable with his people when they welcomed us in late the next afternoon. Familiar talk went on between us, and I felt like they had known me for years. They were kind people, opening their home for us to sleep there that night. Little did we know my family had apparently contacted them earlier, needing to know where their little church cherub was. I was on the wanted list. By now my parents must have felt I had been somehow kidnapped.

My body and mind craved sleep, but around ten o'clock—so early in the night—I heard my father and brother's voices out in the living room. It startled me. I went out to be greeted by worried looks on their faces. "Sylvia," I heard my father's voice say, "we cannot condone what you are doing. You can come back home with your brother and me in the car I only *loaned* you, or your brother and I will take the car and you will be on your own."

I felt the tight coil still wrenching at my gut. There was no way I could turn back. I heard myself respond, "Take the car; we don't need it."

No longer feeling we were wanted in Uncle Max and Aunt Sue's home, we grabbed our bags and left. I felt myself stumbling, attached at the hip to Sam, as we made our way down the street to the main road. We were officially hitchhikers. We were picked up by a Volkswagen bus painted with peace signs on the side. As we got in, the sweet smell of marijuana hit my nostrils. They seemed kind enough and spoke in short, cut-off sentences. I had never been in such a bizarre group, but they did get us—in the chilly darkness of night—to Orangeburg, South Carolina.

I was weary to the bone. I still had enough in my checking account to get us a decent motel room, where we sank in passionate love-making onto an old box-spring mattress. This was not my idea of resting. We were no sooner done when Sam wanted to go back out in the night for something. I followed but could not tell what he was looking for. Then, there it was, a car dealership with a car sitting empty and keys in the ignition. He signaled me to quickly get in, which I did with some trepidation. Were we about to become car thieves in a sable brown 1971 Buick LeSabre?

And this is how our journey would pass for the next six weeks. We would sell a spare tire for gas or food money, or I would write a bad check for a room. Our whole expedition south was in this beautiful *stolen* vehicle. I knew it was wrong, but when I brought it up with Sam, he seemed more amused than guilty. He was so at ease with it, while I looked warily side to side, ahead and behind, for the sight of a police car. By now, I began to sense taking off with this dashing young man may not have been a very good idea, but in my mind it was too late. I was smitten at all costs. We were Bonnie and Clyde, to Sam's thinking, only minus the guns. In my mind we were birds of a feather stealing our way into the South.

The coil still unwinding in me, we went on together. I did not care where this man was coming from, nor did I care where we were going. All I cared about was the closeness and an intimacy I had never before known. I only cared to be with him, to hold onto the first real and personal passion I had ever experienced. In my confused mind, I was in it for the long haul.

Less than forty-eight hours into our expedition, we entered the state of Florida. I remember thinking it was the longest state I had ever gone through. By afternoon we were crossing Alligator Alley and entering a little town called Naples. We drove through the downtown, pulling up at last to the Gulf of Mexico. The sweet scent of ocean water lured us to the edge. We stood gazing out over it, arm in arm, caught in a moment of romance. I think we were both running on pure passion and sex, no two ways about it. We were caught, and we were free.

Soon we were making our way up Fifth Avenue, then Tamiami Trail to the Starlight Motel. A lovely middle-aged woman named Jewel greeted us in the office. I remember thinking how pretty she was, tall with long blonde hair pulled back in a braid. I swallowed my guilt as I made a worthless check out for her. But by now I was starting to feel woozy and hot. Only it was not the weather—I was getting sick.

Sam went out for groceries while I lay writhing on the bed. We ate buttered baloney sandwiches with mustard, downing cold beer between bites. As hungry as I was, I struggled to keep it down. But the food did nothing for my sickness. By seven o'clock that evening, I was burning up with fever. My abdomen felt like it was full of hot coals, and my urine burned me like fire. Sam took me by the hand, helping me to the car. We ended up in the emergency room of the local hospital, where they tested my urine and gave me an antibiotic. I had a bladder infection, and I was supposed to just rest. Well, *that* was not about to happen.

We ended up back at the motel, but by ten o'clock I found myself being drug by the hand back to the LeSabre. We were driving north toward God knows where. I could not believe how restless Sam was. He almost seemed to be chasing his tail. Finally, he made a left turn in the small town of Bonita Springs, down a small access road, and recklessly right out onto the beach. The tires became entrenched in the sand. He spun the wheels only for a few seconds and then dove out onto the beach, yelling at me to help wipe the fingerprints off the car. We were ditching it! I took a small handkerchief out of my pocket and did the best I could, but soon Sam had me by the hand again and we were making our way by foot back down that road to the trail.

We walked and walked. I struggled to get one foot in front of another. I had grown weak. Finally we came to a Holiday Inn where Sam stole at least eight—maybe ten—license plates from the cars of unsuspecting guests. I don't know how many he managed to get into his hands, but then, as we continued our trudge south, back toward Naples, he began throwing the plates to the side of the road. I could not figure out in my feverish head just why he was doing this. He hung onto only one plate. Finally, we made it back to our motel, and I thought surely now we would rest. But we didn't.

Let me tell you, I followed this young man like he was a messiah. I seemed to be his getaway plan. I was hundreds of miles from home, growing weaker by the hour, and tired—so dreadfully tired. I was confused by Sam's behavior. He was taking me on the journey of my life. Where was I? What were we doing? Why? Why, why, why …?

We kept walking down the Trail past a shopping mall, several hotels, and some condominiums. The car dealerships, naturally, were of interest to Sam. Finally we came to a Ford dealership where a lovely little blue Ford Pinto sat, keys in the ignition, outside the service door. They might as well have put his name on it, because without hesitation he took it—and we were out of there!

The rest of our journey took place over six weeks and is kind of a blur in my memory. We drove and drove, up the west coast of Florida, across the panhandle, and into Alabama. North, north, north we drove. I should say Sam drove. I was pretty much just a bystander by now, so gullible. The sky had grown dark with winter. At one point a huge flock of crows flew ominously overhead. I remember feeling so lost. Sam wanted to get to Nashville, but his heart was into wanting to see his brother, Clarence, in the Huntsville, Alabama prison. I began to see where Sam's sadness lie, his sense of needing to keep his family together. I wondered how many thieves he had for brothers. He was proud of one brother who was the mayor of the Borough of Penbrook, just outside Harrisburg.

We drove right past Huntsville, wanting to get to Nashville. But Nashville turned out to be only another progression of bars, dives, and cheap motels. I think we spent more time there than even in Naples, which if I remember correctly was less than twenty-four hours. Sam seemed to like trashing motel rooms too, another thing I could make no sense of at all. He would put the stopper in the sinks of bathrooms, and we would leave with the water running! Every shred of decency in me was screaming, "This is not right!" Twice, at least, we made off with televisions to barter for cash at pawn shops. This would eventually bring our little escapade to an end, but it sustained us for weeks. Still, I clung to Sam's coattails like he had all the answers to what persisted in perplexing me, which was really only my pain and mental confusion.

We drove through Carlisle, Kentucky, where I got a twinge of homesickness, thinking about my grandparents back in Carlisle, Pennsylvania. If I'd had a cell phone, I honestly think I would have phoned home or phoned *someone* at this point. But I didn't, of course, so I kept right on going. My fever and infection had subsided after forty-eight hours. But I was getting just so weak and tired—tired of the running, tired of not eating, and tired, mostly, just of living.

With Tammy Wynette bellowing out, "Stand by your man" over the car radio, Sam cut sharply down, deep into the heart of Texas. I had thought the trek south through Florida a long trip, but the Texas roads seemed even longer. At one point he was sure we would get caught at a sobriety checkpoint. He seemed exceptionally on edge. But somehow we made it through.

We drove up through New Mexico to the only other place foremost on Sam's mind. Like a lot of suckers, he wanted to get rich in Las Vegas. But all we really got was drunk in a lot of casinos and topless bars, plus the usual bars with cheap brew and women. I guess, had I still been a Girl Scout at this point, I would have gotten a merit badge for being a cheap woman. After all, I was really only along for the ride, and of course, the escape.

It is difficult for me to say how many days we were in Las Vegas, because we only slept for two or three hours at a time. One day just melted into the next. I saw the bags under Sam's eyes grow deeper with the wear and tear our expedition was having on him. After Vegas, we drove all the next day just to get to California, only to turn around in San Bernardino and drive back to Nevada for another night of gambling. It was in St. George, Utah, the next morning that our luck—if it was luck that got us there at all—ran out.

We had heisted a really big television at the last motel—we certainly didn't get any sleep! Common sense would tell most people that a big TV in the back of a small hatchback car was a very *big* mistake. The next day we found ourselves followed by several cop cars, sirens blaring and lights flashing, going up and down the streets of St. George, Utah. I felt panic inside while also feeling hope—hope, really, that someone would bring this unreasonable escapade to a reasonable end. Above all, I was exhausted— worn to the bone. By now I had not slept one solid night for close to a month and a half. Yes, it took getting locked up for this little *Bonnie* to stop kicking. I had to get real about where I was going, what I was doing, and who I was with while doing it.

I needed most of all just to put my head down and rest. When Sam finally veered our little Pinto into the parking lot of a small strip mall, I felt I had reached my destination, finally. Sam darted from the car into a Laundromat; I just stood, dazed, beside it. I found myself in handcuffs sitting in a squad car, peering out as they took the love of my life into another car. As usual, I was numb to what was going on around me. As I gazed at him, my heart bled with remorse. Was getting caught my fault?

I was taken to the county lockup, a tiny concrete block cell with a toilet, sink, and concrete slab bed with a thin vinyl mattress. Anyone else would have rested after being through what I had just experienced. Not me; with every ounce of my being, I wanted to be where Sam was, in whatever cell he was in. In my extreme restlessness and agitation, I bounced like a monkey in a cage all over that nine-by-nine cell with a twelve-foot ceiling and fluorescent lights overhead. The placebo of Sam's presence in my life was being challenged. I needed him to live, or so I thought. Someone brought me a few magazines to help get me through the long weekend. I tore several editions of *The Ladies Home Journal* into pictures and the letters to spell, "S-a-m-u-e-l … M-c-Q-u-e-e-n" and glued them with spit balls to the polished concrete walls. I used any means I could to be close to him, if even just in my mind. At night I heard someone tapping out Morse Code on the plumbing from somewhere in the courthouse. I was sure it was him.

On Sunday morning, the Mormon sheriff's wife came to visit me. She seemed concerned. I had barely eaten all weekend, and she was the bearer of news I did not care to hear. She said, "Your mother and father and family love you. They want you home." To this she added, "The Collier County, Florida, sheriff is sending officers to escort you and your young friend back to Naples, where the car you stole came from. Now why don't you eat something to give you strength for the road ahead?" I was thrilled at this piece of information; at least for a while Sam and I would be together again.

That night was even longer than the two nights prior. Someone else was brought into the cell next to mine. I pressed my face against the window of my cell door to get a better look, but all I saw was a bright but barren hallway. The next morning when I was led upstairs and out to a waiting squad car, I felt a surge of newfound energy, an electricity through my somewhat emaciated body. Then, to the delight of my eyes, there sat Sam handcuffed in the seat next to me. Once again my whole body was drawn to him, but with one of the officers staring back at us, all we could do was exchange hungry looks with each other.

I noticed Sam looked thin and tired. My own head felt like a hundred pounds on my stooped shoulders. Yes, we were living on love, but the kind of life we had been living did not love us. I knew what we had been doing was wrong, but inside I felt life owed me something for all the seemingly fruitless effort and pain I had put into it. I had no idea what lay on the road ahead. I didn't want to know. I would take whatever came, as long as this wonderful, devilish young man was still in my life.

The drive back to Florida was long and arduous, longer, it seemed, than the weeks we had traveled all across America. I wanted desperately to move closer to Sam. Inhibition once again choked me. The dark side of me that had been released so freely with him was once again subdued. When we stopped to eat an hour into the trip, I teetered and almost fell getting out of the car. I was weak as a runt. One officer put his arm out to keep me from falling, but I righted myself instantly. This final leg of the journey was getting to be just a bit too much, but I was young and innately strong. My hamburger and fries were prepared well enough, but it just tasted like cardboard to me. Nothing was the same. I was a prisoner—and yet I still felt a kind of release. There was no more tight coil in me.

That night I was placed in an Albuquerque jail where the accommodations were more like a Nazi concentration camp—no food, not even a toilet or water. I held myself as long as I could, pacing most of the night, and finally I went to piss in the little privy hole to the rear of the cell. I thought morning would never come. But it did, along with another long, long day of travel. I peered out the window as the driver sped over mile after mile of, once again, barren, flat Texas roads.

Finally, we arrived in Naples, and I felt like I had come home. But once again Sam and I were locked in separate cells. This time my cell was about eighty feet by twenty feet, packed with roughly thirty women. It was crowded, sweaty, and dirty. There was not even a bunk on which to lay my head down. I slept on the floor with a blanket, using my arm for a pillow. As I wept quietly to myself, a woman of maybe forty-five years old, a trustee working at the jail, must have heard me. She came to the outside of the bars and tried in a tender, womanly way to comfort me. Her name was Rochelle, and I would meet her later at the hospital where she was working as a nurse's aide. An eighteen-year-old girl named Pancake who spoke with a childlike voice seemed to want to make friends. She had a toddler son she missed; we all missed someone. I grew weary quickly of these accommodations. But I would have rather they had locked me up and thrown away the key than what happened next.

The following morning I was brought out to the brightly lit courthouse station, where officers and clerks were busily going about their workday. I was led to a small conference room with a table and a few chairs. There sat my mother and father, their faces full of the stress and grief. The circumstances were strange to us. Father was on my left, Mother on his left. In a severe voice I heard Mother say, "Sylvia, what are ... you ... doing?"

Immediately I leaned toward Father, imploring him, "Father, tell Mother to please shut up, will you? And will you tell me, what am I supposed to do? I love Sam, and I need to be with him." My parents were trying to talk sense into me. Later, their attorney, Mr. Hadcock, did the same while also chastising me for being so foolish. But what could be foolish about the feelings I had for Sam?

After a week in the cramped Collier County Prison, I was released on bail. And much to my surprise, so was Sam. Father, bless his heart, wanted me to be happy. Had he connected with me thoroughly, he would have realized the kind of blind passion behind our insane behaviors and that it would lead to more poor decisions on my part. I think he somehow sensed how much I detested Mother's controlling manner. I knew she meant well, but she had a way about her that made me so furious. He and Mother may have both blamed themselves for my rash, unseemly behavior. Maybe they suffered from a kind of deep parental *guilt* having focused so intensely on the business over the years, that now I was expressing a sense of abandonment. Anyway, this is what I was feeling.

I could not even look at Mother that morning in the conference room. Should I be feeling guilty? I didn't think so. But I did. That did not stop me from what happened next. Mind you, I was still without brakes.

In an effort to find connections in the Naples area, Mother and Father had called on the pastor of a local Presbyterian church. They no doubt told him of my irrational behavior but that I had been their little cherub back home. In response he connected them with a parishioner's home where I could board while awaiting a hearing. With their encouragement, I went to the community hospital for gainful employment. However, none of us were aware of just how toxic this kind of work was for me. But there I was, the honorable, hardworking little nurse. We were all working hard to show the local authority what a good girl I really was, while inside—inside my dark being, where all I could feel was depression and pessimism—I stewed and stormed.

> *Wheel going around and around, clicking, spinning, driving me further into life, away from, toward. Where have I begun, where have I been, where am I going? I just keep pedaling, around and around ... I saw what I saw, I see what I see, I will see what there is to see. Oh, wheel going around and around, clicking, spinning, driving me further, further, further ... When I stop, nobody knows; where I stop I know not either. I just am, I just am, I ... just ... am. I ... am ... I am ... I ... I ... I ... am ... am ... am ...*

But there was no real sense of connection to the real truth. That would happen twenty-six years later, long after my parents departed from this life. At this point, though, we were all blinded and confused by what was happening to us. I have no idea how Sam found a home to stay in. Both of us were awaiting our court appearances.

Sam's rooming house was on the outskirts of town. I know because it barely took an hour after my parents left for me to find him. He called, or I called. I don't recall the details, only the magnetism between us. We were drawn like ships in the night, our radar peaked and ready to carouse. We spent the day rolling in lust in his bed at the house while the owner's teen and adolescent kids smoked pot in the living room. I remember because they offered me a joint, but something inside told me not to add that to my list of "new experiences." That evening is when all hell broke loose in the peaceful little town of Naples and thereabout.

Sam and I were hopping from bar to bar on foot, becoming disgustingly inebriated until around ten o'clock that evening. Maybe you can guess what happened next. We came out of a bar along the Gordon River, and next thing you know, I was sitting next to Sam in another stolen car! I could tell he was agitated. He wanted out of town, any place but where we were facing felony charges and prison time. He knew it, and I knew it. Next thing I remember is once again being chased by police cars up North Tamiami Trail. Again he swerved into a mall parking lot, diving and running into the dark night. A gunshot rang out. I just stood there in a horrified stupor. Nothing of our behavior made sense to me, but there I was in the thick of it. The evening ended at a police station. I was in such a blackout I do not remember getting back to the house.

Wheel going around and around …

By now Mother and Father were back in Pennsylvania, but I did get a call from Father the next morning. He expressed to me, "Sylvia, you made your bed, now lie in it!" With that he hung up. I don't think I had ever heard him so angry. The woman, who had so graciously allowed me to stay in her home, reneged. I was forced to move to a small bungalow on the outskirts of town, staying with young Pancake and two other women. One evening I was moved to call home to check whether I had yet been disowned.

I walked about a half mile up the road to find a phone booth. It was dark, and I looked up into the deepest, bluest, starriest night sky I could ever remember seeing. The lights of the Marco Island Bridge were in the distance. The booth was outside a restaurant where people were inside happily dining with friends and family. I had a bout of intense loneliness. I had no sooner stepped inside to call when, to my horror, I realize the light had drawn hundreds of chameleons. It must have looked like a Charlie Chaplin movie, because I jumped backward to get out as fast as I had stepped in. I had to dial and speak with the cord at its fullest length to avoid an encounter with the bizarre little specimens warming themselves on the glass.

I rented a bicycle and rode ten miles into the hospital and back for work. Somehow it did not seem far, since the terrain was so flat. I barely felt the ride. And the salty, warm sea air refreshed me by the time I got back in the evening. In less than a week my dear father and *fix-it* mother somehow arranged with the judge, since the whole episode was so out of character for me, to have the charges dropped. But there was one proviso—I was to return to Pennsylvania to finish nursing school at the Polyclinic Hospital. It was not a choice; it was a demand. My family also wanted me back in the choir; this was simply understood. However, nothing in me wanted to sing. I was dying inside, but nobody knew this side of me. My real time of reckoning was years to come. And oh, did it come.

I only continued to work on a surgical floor of the hospital for another week until it was time to fly back to my home state. I did so with great sadness; I was leaving behind the one true love I had ever had. Sam was convicted of multiple felonies and sentenced to years in prison. This was far from his first encounter with the law. I never got all the details, but I believe the state of Florida got first dibs on him, and then Pennsylvania, which could have meant more prison time. Still, I wanted to wait for him to get out so we could marry and have a life together. I just could not get it through my head that he was irresponsible, irascible, and downright bad news. I felt like I was going home to my own kind of prison. I had no desire to finish nursing—not really. It only meant more years of suffering. But what could I do? I had to act like the little goodie two shoes I had been portrayed to be.

It was a sunny day in February when my plane touched down at our airport in Middletown. However, inside me it was darkness and foreboding.

It may as well have been raining dead ducks, because that was how I felt. The whole family was there to greet me like I had been on vacation in Europe. I felt really ashamed of myself now, for the first time. What had I done to this wonderful family, the people who loved me and prayed for my return? I believe my parents had told my grandparents I was visiting friends in Florida or some other acceptable yarn. For the first time, too, I even considered getting in touch with the young Columbian man, Alfonso, who had pursued me since high school. I had visions of myself getting off a plane in Bogota, wearing a navy blue nurse's cape and Polyclinic graduate's cap, proud as a peacock and ready to be his bride. I was such a dreamer.

I soon found myself back in the old, loudly reverberating halls of the nursing school dorm, toting books and notepads from classroom to clinic and back to the dorm. It was surreal. The popular song that blared from a radio down the hall was "Sylvia's Mother Says." Well, Mother had *said*, and there I was, living her dream, not mine. I hated every moment I was there. Then, the unthinkable happened—Hurricane Agnes came through our area.

It rained solid the whole month of June 1972. The river overflowed upon the whole uptown area. All of Greater Harrisburg was inundated, and our hospital was like an island. No one could get in, nor could anyone leave. We were expected to help staff the hospital. I found myself once again working as a kind of nurse technician—running the concrete floors, lifting huge patients, and running the stairwells due to the elevators being flooded. Someone even had to carry meals up several flights of stairs. Patients, if they were able, lined up cafeteria-style for meals. The worst thing, I thought, was the lack of ventilation due to being on auxiliary power. The workers and professionals unfortunate enough to be stuck there slept in empty rooms or on cots in utility areas.

With all this going on, we were still expected to study and pass exams. As usual I quickly burned out. It would be just a matter of time until I would be out of there again. The walls of my room came in on me, more of the same long nightmare. I panicked every evening when I came back to my room. I kept the windows open in spite of the horrible oil and exhaust fumes. Noisy choppers flew constantly overhead. I was living Dante's Paradise Lost. I was lost. But my heart was what hurt the most. Sam was in Florida in prison, and I was thousands of miles away, pretending to be the nurse.

> *Wheel going around and around, clicking, spinning,*
> *driving me further into life, away from, toward. Where*
> *have I begun, where have I been, where am I going?*

When the waters had parted and the sun shone once again, I was again out of that place. I was a prisoner enough; why ask for more walls and more aggravation in my life? So for the rest of that summer I was free to be me, at least to some extent. I had no idea who that person—Sylvia—really was. I was still under my mother's thumb, bowing to her every whim and fancy. I helped out in the mail-order business, still in our basement. But oh how I wished I could wake to my own time clock instead of my mother's, "Yoohoo … Sylvia … it's time to get up …" at seven o'clock on a Saturday morning. Didn't she know I was old enough to take some responsibility for my life? If only she could let me think for myself. I needed that so badly.

All that Summer I rode with the Harrisburg Bicycle Club. I always felt so free on my *wheel*. And it was a chance to meet new people and, possibly, I hoped to get some idea where I was going next in my life. I needed a transplant, to get away to some place where I could be myself. But was there such a place? Could I really live on my own? Inside I had such doubts about myself. And deep inside me lingered thoughts of that young man I had left down in a Florida prison. He had nobody there for him, and there I was surrounded by people who loved me and really cared about me. I just could not accept their love freely, nor could I any longer accept the free room and board. A transplant was exactly what I needed. But this time it had to be of my own choosing, with my own energy and drive.

One of the members of the bicycle club was a seventy-five-year-old man named Ed Mood who had at the age of seventy-four rode his bicycle, a blue, three-speed Raleigh just like mine, from Pennsylvania to Florida. Just the thought took my breath away; to think that someone his age could ride that far! He planted a seed of an idea in my mind. For the next two months, I spent every spare moment taking my bicycle apart, oiling and lubing it, and changing a flat. I took a large piece of green canvas I found lying around the house and made saddle bags for it. I quietly planned, my second getaway imminent. For the first time, I felt real hope. Even a prayer welled up inside me, "God, can I do this? Please help me to make this trip."

On the evening of Thursday, August 5, Father saw me standing at the edge of the carport, looking longingly up at a plane as it flew silently by, way up in the sky. He came and stood next to me and said with such tenderness, "Sylvia, you're thinking of leaving again, aren't you?"

If I could be honest with anyone at this point, it had to be him, the way he bailed me out and kept bailing me out financially. "Yes, Father, I do. I have to go somewhere—any place but here. I have to get away." I could have added, "away from Mother," but I didn't. He knew.

I still hung onto myself in the image of a nurse. I wanted to fulfill that dream for myself because it did make me feel I could do something real in life—make people *feel* better. I was good, at least, at talking people out of feeling bad. I also loved the feeling of intimacy I had with patients when I was giving a bed bath or rubbing a back. I didn't think I was cut out for anything else. So, hesitating inside, not knowing if I could even make a trip on a bicycle to Florida, I prayed, "God, if you want me to do this, you will have to give me some sort of sign." I had heard there was a good nursing school in Columbia, North Carolina, so I conjured up a little fib. I told my family I was aiming to settle there to finish nursing school. I knew if I told them I was thinking of riding to Florida, they would lock me up and throw away the key.

"Sleep to Night" in

Slumberland MOTEL

"MODERN AS AMERICA"

2 MILES NORTH ON U.S. 301 Orangeburg, S. C.

GOING MY WAY

Finally, on the morning of August 7, the backseat and trunk of another of Father's old delivery cars, even the front seat, were packed to the hilt with my belongings. Mounted on the back was my blue, three-speed Raleigh bicycle. After hugs, kisses, and wishes for good luck, I drove down the driveway, leaving everybody waving me off. I again took off down Route 15, this time alone. But in my heart my only destination was a prison in Florida and maybe Gainesville where I knew there was a community college for nursing studies. I was scared inside—really scared. I had never done anything like this on my own, but I knew if I was to ever get a sense of my own person, of who I really was, I had to do it.

Again the miles clicked by, this time daylight hours, and I had a plan. No more relying on a young man who was obviously not in his right mind. Then again, neither had I been even remotely sane. But how else was I going to learn? How was I going to get anywhere in life if I could not learn to think for myself, be self-sufficient, and be fiscally responsible? Just like the last time, I drove practically nonstop, but this time I wanted only to get to where Sam and I first stole a car: Orangeburg, South Carolina. By then, I figured, I would no doubt have the sign from God I was depending on. I was three miles out from that little town when my sign came; the car broke down.

I called the only foreign car place in the area to tow me: Bozo's Foreign Car Dealership and Repair. I kid you not, that was the name I found in the phone book. I waited restlessly around their small-town shop for a quote of necessary repairs. To my horror, it was three hundred dollars. I froze. I only had that much to get me to Florida and get settled. My first big decision was upon me. But it was not a difficult one; I knew what I had to do. I asked the man if I could pay to store the car and all my belongings behind his fence, and I told him I would send him the three hundred dollars, "down the road." I took off on my bicycle to find the Slumberland Motel where Sam and I had stayed. But this time it was just me, no Sam, no feeling of being driven to do anything unnatural like the last time. I slept like a baby that night. I was nervous, yes, but confident God was with me and would stay with me the whole journey … by wheel, my very own *wheel*.

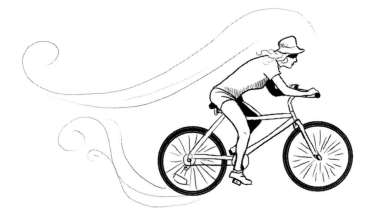

*Wheel going around and around, clicking, spinning, driving
me further into life, away from, toward. Where have I
begun, where have I been, where am I going? I just keep
pedaling, around and around ... I saw what I saw, I see
what I see, I will see what there is to see. Oh, wheel going
around and around, clicking, spinning, driving me further,
further, further ... When I stop, nobody knows; where I
stop I know not either. I just am, I just am, I ... just ... am.
I ... am ... I am ... I ... I ... I ... am ... am ... am ...*

I believe I may have ridden twenty or thirty miles that first full day on the road, destination: Florida. I admit I was quite scared. Never had I ventured quite so far from home on a bicycle and all by myself. I had with me an old felt man's hat, under which I carefully tucked my shoulder-length blonde hair in an attempt to look masculine. Surely no one would bother a young man traveling solo down a main road, but a woman? I just did not know what to expect from passersby. There were many long, lonely stretches of road ahead. During those first few miles, I was reminded of John Bunyan's allegory, *Pilgrim's Progress,* our tenth-grade homeroom teacher had read to us.

As the wheels spun beneath me, the gears steadily clicking ... *click, click, click, click* ... I became Christian in the book, fleeing the City of Destruction ... *click, click, click, click.* I had left my hometown in a desecrated state ... *click, click, click, click.* I had invested so much hope ... *click, click, click, click* ... into the trip, the journey ... *click, click, click, click* ... down that southern road. The south wind blew into my face ... *click, click, click, click* ... and the Spanish Moss ... *click, click, click, click* ... swung from the tall oaks ... *click, click, click, click* ... to the side of the road ... *click, click, click, click* ... I had always thought of myself ... *click, click, click, click* ... as a Christian ... *click, click, click, click.* It was the way we were raised ... *click, click, click, click* ... I had trouble, however ... *click, click, click, click* ... with the concept that Jesus suffered and died on the cross to save me ... *click, click, click, click* ... It was hard living ... *click, click, click, click* ... with so much physical pain and feeling saved. I longed to know ... *click, click, click, click* ... the real truth of Christ being hung on that tree ... *click, click, click, click* ...

If I was saved … *click, click, click, click* … why was I so miserable all the time? *Click, click, click, click* … Where was Jesus in my suffering? I always … *click, click, click, click* … seemed to go the extra mile at my work … *click, click, click, click* … and in making my family happy … *click, click, click, click* … but all it ever seemed to get me … *click, click, click, click* … was more suffering. I was a seeker of truth … *click, click, click, click* … that was the real gist of my trip. Perhaps … *click, click, click, click* … God would reveal himself to me in a new way … *click, click, click, click* … something like he did with Moses and the burning bush … *click, click, click, click* … the water from a rock … *click, click, click, click* … or manna from heaven. I was young … *click, click, click, click* … ideal, and … *click, click, click, click* … open to answers, new insights … *click, click, click, click* …

When the evening of my first day on the road was upon me, I had a plan. I would stop at a motel where there were people around and try to get to know them a little. Then, after everyone went into their respective motel rooms, I would find someplace nearby, hopefully well lit, where I could rest in the shadow of a tree. That way, were I to need help during the night, I would at least have doors to knock on, or at the very least ears to pierce with my screams. I hoped it would not come to that. Just as the August sun began to set, I found the perfect place.

I came to a motel where there was an elderly couple from Deerfield Park, Florida. They were swinging on the glider on the cool, grassy lawn out front. It was relaxing to just sit and talk to them, and they were interested in my travel plans. I got their address and promised to try to find them when I got to their town in southeast Florida. All too soon, though, they were telling me good night and going into their room. I dawdled back a bit but soon slipped to the rear of the motel, where there was a good, bright searchlight directed into a wooded area. I lay on a blanket in the shadow of a tree, tarp on top of me. But I barely got a wink of sleep. I just felt too exposed, in harm's way. I realized I could not do this every night. Sure, I could rest some this way, but I would have to get some sleep eventually.

On the second day, I was up before the sun, riding, riding, riding … A long road lay ahead. I was tired from my trip the day before, but I was still gung-ho, ready to go. God knew I had had much more tiresome days before, the days I had worked relentlessly at the hospital when pain was all I knew. This was not painful, at all. Bicycling was one activity—unlike running—that did not leave me in the suffering mode. The longer I was on the road and the further I got, however, I had a different kind of pain—butt pain. By the time I got to southeast Florida I had towels and extra clothing wrapped around the bicycle seat to soothe my bottom. Even this pain, however, was nothing compared to what I had experienced working those months at the hospital across the river or those years at Polyclinic Hospital as a student.

I was blessed—these roads, the people I met on the roads, a life to call my own, and the excitement of a new life ahead of me. I had a good breakfast for two or three bucks in the morning and a bosom full of hope to speed me down those open, free roads. *Click, click, click, click, click, click ...* The sound of my wheels beneath me was so soothing. I had written my family from Orangeburg, but I gave no clue I was taking off by bicycle. I lied a lot to them, but I felt I had to protect myself and separate my thoughts from theirs. I even told them I had driven all over Columbia, North Carolina, where I was supposedly going to settle and go back to nursing school. I would say anything to appease my mother. I think up until I left on my own I was mostly like the character, Pliable, in *Pilgrim's Progress*. I just wanted people to be happy, so I would say anything to this end. I surely had a lot of maturing to do—really a lot.

The second night was spent in Statesboro, Georgia. I swore this was the nicest little town I had ever been in. As I rode into town ... *click, click, click, click ...* I could hear a baseball game going on at a nearby ball field. The houses were big, gabled, and two story, many with wraparound porches and rocking chairs. The first thing I did was find a Laundromat to get some of the sweat out of my few clothing articles. Plus, this was a good place just to be around people and have friendly conversations. I took a bath in the sink of a gas station restroom. As the sun began to fall below the western horizon I located a remote place among some trees in the city park. However, sleep evaded me again.

The next night I had to find a cheap motel to get some sleep. Over the next four weeks, I found motels for as little as seven or nine dollars a night. I would always take my bicycle into the room with me. I don't think I even had a lock or chain. Occasionally I stopped for two nights to give my body a chance to revive. When I got to Jessup, Georgia, I got the idea to name my little blue Raleigh Jesse, like it was a mule I was riding. I knew in the back of my mind I would have to eventually tell my family what I was doing, but I was in no hurry. The very next day I got the idea to send a postcard home, telling everybody of my adventure ... and on a *mule*, too.

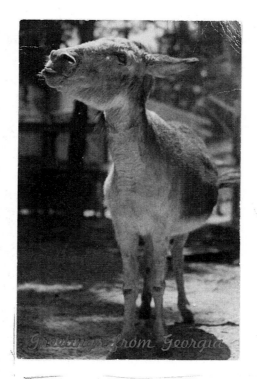

Postcard of Maud (Jesse) the Mule
The Famous *Kissing Jackass*
Courtesy of Mackey's Animal Farm
Richmond Hill, GA
(twenty-three miles south of Savannah, U.S. Rt.17)

August 12, 1972

Dear Mother, Father, and Wendy, the going is mighty slow. No mechanical problems except for an occasional stop—to tie a shoe (Ω). *We have put 200.9 miles on the odometer since Orangeburg, South Carolina. The only thing that hurts is my seat* (and Jesse's back, but she never complains).

Finally, one day at the southernmost edge of Georgia, I was going through a little borough named Carlisle. And just as it was with Sam when we passed through Carlisle, Kentucky, this triggered an extreme bout of homesickness in me. I found a brick structure marked Bell Telephone Company, so I thought I would go in to make my first call home. To my disappointment, it was only a terminal building, and all I had was a payphone on an outside wall to make the call.

Byron answered. I remember fear welling up inside me. I detested his constant talk and punning at home, but now—well, now I just wanted him to go on talking, filling my lonely heart with his mindless babble. It didn't seem so mindless anymore. He was so far away. Then Mother and Father came on the extension phones. They expressed their extreme concern, but they also praised me for my courage. The love and compassion they shared with me fueled the whole rest of the journey that day. After meatloaf and mashed potatoes for dinner that evening, I slept like I had been walloped on the head with a tree branch. The dreams were sweet.

One very frightening part of the journey—besides the everyday experience of lonely road and fast-passing cars—was going through Okefenokee Swamp. It was miles and miles of barren road, with only the tall pine trees on either side. I passed one little log cabin with a skinny, little old black lady in a rocking chair on the porch. Either she did not see me or she saw me as the enemy, because she did not return my wave and hello. My mind grew frantic the further I got into the swamp. Very few cars even passed me. I thought to myself, *What if some guy in a car stops and approaches me? I would be a sitting duck for abduction.* Thank God, like a lot of fears, nothing came of this one either.

One of the advantages of traveling by bicycle as opposed to motor vehicles is I was able to stop, breathe in the fresh air, and take in the scenery. It was thrilling—very, *very* thrilling. I remember stopping on the small two-lane bridge that crossed the Suwanee River. There I stood humming a few bars of Stephen Foster's "Way Down upon the Suwanee River, far, far away ..." This was so real. The whole experience was something I knew I would never forget. Life was real, I was real, and, for the first time in a long time, I was genuinely happy. I would soon, however, have to face one of the reasons I was in Florida again—my ill-begotten boyfriend, Sam.

I did not know in what state of being I would find him as I made my way toward Raiford Prison. It was a big, brick structure with razor-sharp barbed wire spanning the whole outside perimeter. The place almost seemed abandoned as I approached, but once I was inside and cleared for visitation, I was not ready for what I was about to observe. Sam resisted visiting with me. He did not want anything to do with me, at least overtly. I sensed, however, his despondency had to do with how different our circumstances were. He was not free. I wanted to show him love and affection but was met by chilly indifference. This, I knew, was not the real Sam. But then again, did I even know the real Sam? The visit was over in less than ten minutes. I cried as I walked back to my bicycle. Why did I even bother? It just seemed to bring him more pain.

My next point of interest was Gainesville because I knew there was a community college there where I might finish *my nursing*. I just wanted to finally wrap up this elusive goal; whether I liked nursing or not, I wanted to "qualify" somehow. I still held onto the thought that nursing was my destiny. I got to this pleasant little college town by 8:00 a.m. the next day. The students were busily walking from college building to college building, or lingering with friends under the many majestic oak boughs. After only one or two hours of meandering through the relatively quiet streets, I knew this was not where I belonged. *Click, click, click, click …*

> *Wheel going around and around, clicking, spinning, driving me further into life, away from, toward. Where have I begun, where have I been, where am I going? I just keep pedaling, around and around … I saw what I saw, I see what I see, I will see what there is to see. Oh, wheel going around and around, clicking, spinning, driving me further, further, further … When I stop, nobody knows; where I stop I know not either. I just am, I just am, I … just … am. I … am … I am … I … I … I … am … am … am …*

I turned to my little road map to find the next point of interest. I knew right away. I pointed my wheel east and rode mightily for Hawthorne, Florida. I had no "e" on the end of my last name, Hawthorn, but surely a town of this name would hold some meaning for me. Well, it didn't.

In fact, for want of a simple traffic light at the center of town or a voice from heaven saying, "Sylvia, you are in Hawthorne," I almost missed the town completely. I did find a little antique store at the edge of town, filled with items mostly from Scranton, Pennsylvania. An old copy of Rachael Carson's *The Sea around Us* in hand, I stretched out on top of my blanket on a cool patch of green grass and soaked up her beautiful words. I felt such a sense of peace and unusual belonging. Yes, even in this faraway place I felt I was a part of the land beneath me. Then I scratched out a postcard to home.

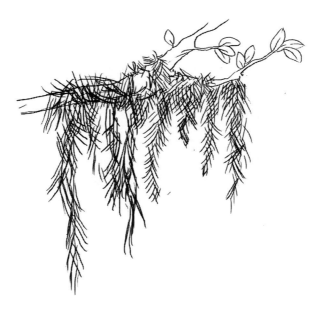

Wednesday August 16, 1972

Dear Mother, Father, and Wendy,

I am stretched out on the lawn of an antique dealer, Mr. Williams. Much of his merchandise is from Scranton, Pennsylvania. As perhaps you will see by the postmark, this place is about a quarter-mile outside the little town of Hawthorne. I've just finished a picnic lunch of honey bread and orange juice, and now I'm reading from Rachel Carson's book, *The Sea around Us*. The book is practically falling apart, so as I read a few pages, I take them out and send them to Sam. Hasn't God given us a beautiful earth? Even the hills have become my friends. God bless you.

Love,

Sylvia

Feeling unusually revived from my little siesta, I packed up my gear and purchase and decided, *I want to go to the sea.* I rode and rode and rode … *click, click, click, click* … through the night. I was glad for my little generator light attached to the front wheel. It made just enough light to see that dark road unfold in front of me. I grew weary but continued my journey, pedaling almost frantically. I didn't care. All I cared about was getting to the ocean. Just as the sun was rising, I came to a small but glorious little park. The sunlight caught droplets of dew as they left their rainbows on my weary, excited mind. I felt or sensed if I just keep pedaling there would be a pot of gold on the other side of these woods. Maybe it was a figment of my imagination, but it felt real. Everything was real—*scary* and real. In fact, it was so scary I could have died right then and been happy.

By about ten that next morning, I saw it—the Atlantic Ocean. I was in Flagler Beach, Florida. I must mention one of the miracles about this trip on my little three-speed Raleigh bicycle. I had not even one flat tire the whole trip. In fact, it was here in Flagler that I had what I thought might be my first mechanical failure. My front wheel was pushing hard, and I heard a different sound. To my relief, I realized the light generator had clicked on by accident. That was all it was. I mean, I would have known how to change the tire had it been flat, but it wasn't … and I didn't. I smile to myself right now when I think of my good fortune throughout this whole trip. Somebody was with me. Maybe—no, in fact, probably—the prayers of my family had something to do with it. I remember often thinking to myself, *Divine Providence is with me.* There was something bigger out there. The stars must have been lined up perfectly, because something felt right.

I walked my bicycle out onto a boardwalk at Flagler Beach. The sun beat down on my deepening tan. I stood gazing for a few moments but once again turned my wheel south, this time on Route A1A. At this point, I thought little about the hills of my home state of Pennsylvania. The flat terrain and my increased stamina allowed me many more miles than I was used to. I sailed down that coast with such ease, as if there were a big hand at my back pushing me. My next letter home was a long one from Merritt Island.

A sunny Saturday, August 19, 1972

Dear Family,

I miss you, but I can truly say I am enjoying this excursion. I arrived here at Melbourne at 7:30 p.m. Friday, scorched +3 red cyan (a color indicator Father used in his photo lab back home) and tired after a seventy-mile ride. I flopped into bed at about 8:00 p.m. and slept solid until 8:00 this morning. This is the Doumar Court, a nice little place and quite inexpensive, as it is still off season. I'll relax here for a day to cool off and leave early tomorrow morning when the sun is not so hot.

The south wind has been my biggest obstacle, but at times even that is a blessing—so cool ... Yesterday I pulled over to the side of the road beneath some palm trees and gazed out over the Indian River to Merritt Island and the Cape Kennedy Space Center. What a beautiful sight!

This morning after breakfast I rested in a shady park along the river (frogs leaping out of the water), visited the library (the librarians were real nice), and went to the post office. Mother, I stopped at one home where I saw a yellow cat very much like Rusty (her cat), posed like a statue on the porch. He wasn't as friendly as Rusty, but he did enjoy licking the breakfast jelly off my fingers. An elderly lady came out of the house. She seemed to enjoy hearing about my journey, and she wanted to know why I call my bike Jesse. I told her, "Because it's slow as a mule." She laughed.

Wendy, I hope you're well and happy. I guess it won't be long until school begins again, and you'll have plenty of time to be with your friends. Sometimes I wish I were back in high school. It's a happy time.

It may seem to you that I, your oldest daughter and sister, have turned-out to be a "bicycle bum." However, I assure you I have plans, and as they unfold, I'll let you in on them.

For now it is only God and I working it out together. God
bless you.
Love,
Sylvia

PS: From my heart I give thee joy,
I was once a barefoot boy!
All too soon these feet must hide
In the prison cells of pride,
Lose the freedom of the sod,
Like a colt's for work be shod.

—"The Barefoot Boy"
John Greenleaf Whittier

By five o'clock the next day I made it to Juno, just north of Palm
Beach—127 miles of wind-in-the-face riding. I wrote another three-page
letter home. Inside I felt excitement building in me, like I was on the last
leg of my journey south. In my heart I just wanted to get to Naples. In my
head, I wanted to get to Fort Myers, another college town. I will soon reveal
which won, my head or my heart. I wrote to my sister this time.

10:30 Sunday night, August 20, 1972

Dear Wendy,
Hello, Sister, how are you? Today I rode a hundred miles
to get to Jupiter Inlet and Juno Beach. Have you ever seen
a hot coal in a fire? The outside is white, and the inside
glows red. That's what I look like. My hair is turning white
blonde from the sun, and my skin is brown, bordering on
red. I even feel as warm and snug as a coal tucked in this
bed here at the Ranchland Motel.
Do you know what crazy thing I did yesterday? I rode forty
miles before breakfast and then ate two breakfasts, mmm.
I had sixteen ounces of milk, eight ounces of orange juice,
two cups of coffee, and eight donuts. It was delicious fuel!
Maybe it wasn't such a crazy thing riding so far before
breakfast. It saved me from a few hours of hot sun, and the
south wind was not so strong in my face.

After breakfast I rode a sixty-mile stretch without stopping, except for an occasional glug of water. Actually, I had planned to stop after forty more miles (at the eighty-mile mark on my odometer). However, at that point in the trip there was nothing but dry, hot road in the middle of Jonathan Dickinson State Park. As you can imagine, it was a real blessing to arrive at Juno Beach.

There is one more incident, rather sad, that happened on my journey today. A young fellow went roaring by me at ninety miles per hour in his new Corvair convertible. I think he was trying to show off by laying rubber on the road. Instead, when he was done there was not much of anything left on the road except glass. I really felt sorry for the fellow and asked God to settle whatever livewire there was in him to do such a thing. He was lucky to be able to walk away from the wreckage, which was wrapped around a telephone pole. To make matters worse, it all happened right in front of a motel swimming pool, where people witnessed the whole folly.

Tonight I had to ride eight miles into North Palm Beach just to find a fairly inexpensive place to eat. The wind was in my face all the way, just as it was for the last twenty miles of today's journey. I reassured myself that the eight miles of the return to the motel would not be so difficult because the wind would be at my tail. However, by the time I got back on the road to return, a new weather front was bringing wind from the opposite direction!

After getting back from supper, I went into the Hitching Rail Saloon where they had a good music box. There were a few regular old time patrons, so it was really a very quiet place. I ordered one-drink, as it seemed the thing to do when you are in a place like that. It was called a screwdriver, and it was mostly orange juice. While there I met and very cautiously conversed with a man who reminded me of Mr. Hadcock, my lawyer from Naples, only much older. He was good company. We did some laughing, and we talked about the houses he builds, the art of being of service to others, trust, and of course, bicycling. The motel manager was nearby in the office. He came in and introduced himself to everybody as my daddy. I just smiled, but I think one man nearby believed him! The manager was kind in acting the way he did, as it was a rather protective gesture. He knew I was there alone and not 100 percent secure.

I ended my conversation with the gentleman at 9:00, when he got to rattling on about his tropical fish and bird collections. He wanted me to go out turtle egg hunting. I very politely excused myself to come to my room and watch the Leonardo de Vinci special on television.

The special is a continuation from last Sunday evening. Did you see it? DaVinci was brilliant, wasn't he? He was strong and creative. It seems he spent most of his time alone, studying nature. I, too, have learned that being alone brings you close to nature. It's beautiful and complex, but it's worth every quiet and God-given moment you can spend with it.

I must admit, I miss you. Tomorrow I'll get to the entrance of Alligator Alley, and Tuesday morning I leave from there with the wind at my tail all the way west, through Naples and then north to Fort Myers. It will be good to arrive at my destination and make new acquaintances. I'll stay there, work, and perhaps take a course or two at Edison Junior College.

Honestly, Wendy, this trip has me feeling full of vigor and like a young person—as young as you, light and feathery, with a beautiful life ahead and so much to do—to find out—goodness to spread. Do you know what I mean? Good night.

Love,
Sylvia

P.S. (10:50 p.m.) I just made a phone call to "Daddy" manager to report the tide is coming into my room. The rug is wet, and the bathroom shower is leaking—drip, drip. He was nice about it. Zzzzzzz ... I obviously did not care that much.

> **A moment of reflection:** Throughout this entire trip I was driven like Christian in *Pilgrim's Progress* to escape the wreckage of my hometown, but I was probably also looking to escape the feeling my life was wreckage too. The mysterious pain in my chest, along with the spasms around my face and head, gave me the distinct feeling there was something *wrong* with me. Not only that, I could not easily put music, words, and rhythm together with much success. As was apparent from my high school musical days, I was even worse at coordinating choreographic movements. Oh sure, I was a great dancer, but only in free form. All told I felt like the least practical, least coordinated young person that walked this earth. So, even though I so often tried to achieve scholarly accomplishment, I *just couldn't do it!* I talked the talk, continually reassuring my parents I would finish training as a nurse, but I could not walk the walk. I was strangely inept, wounded to the core.

I lingered a few days between Juno Beach and Deerfield Beach. I actually got lost one day as I meandered through the development where the elderly couple lived I had met at the motel that first night of my journey. I remember actually panicking, unable to get back to the main road. I never did find the nice couple. After that I decided not to get off the beaten path again. After all, that is what happened to *Christian* when he met *Mr. Worldly Wiseman* in Pilgrim's Progress—he was nearly crushed by a cliff on the way to *Mr. Legality's* house in the *City of Morality*. Yes, Sylvia, no more getting side tracked.

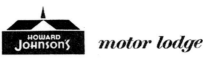

LICENSEE

August 23, 1972

Dear Grandpa,

Hello, Grandpa. How are you? Are your ears mature (i.e., is the corn ripening)? Are the crickets singing to you, "Happy birthday to you, happy birthday to you …"? Hello, Grandma. I love you. It's been three weeks now since we visited. Grandma, would you please give Grandpa a big birthday kiss for me?

Presently, I am resting in a motel in Fort Lauderdale, Florida. The Republican National Convention is on TV. The place where I am is very close to a Seminole Indian Reservation on the Big Cypress Swamp. I arrived here yesterday evening very tired but happy. I have been riding for two weeks since my car broke down in South Carolina. When they fix it, I will come north again, possibly by train. When my journey ends tomorrow in Fort Myers, I'll have ridden nearly a thousand miles.

It is thundering and storming now. Storms are frequent here as two-weather fronts—one from the Gulf and one from the Atlantic—collide over the swampland. Tomorrow I'll ride my last one hundred miles, mostly through barren swamp. My Raleigh three-speed bicycle still shines like new, she coasts like new, and I've not had a single flat tire (though I'm prepared for it if she does). With the wind I go twenty mph.

The hospitality on my journey has been wonderful. People are kind. They direct me to good places to stay. I've had offers to rest in people's homes. They want to hear all about my travels. They also direct me to the best routes to travel.

Grandpa, bicycle travel is the new, clean, quiet, and upcoming means of travel in the future. People are learning their own capacity to move. It's beautiful, and the more of us who set the example—by riding and walking—the faster we will learn. When I talk with other travelers and with the townspeople, many of them are pleased with the idea of cross-country cycling, while others gasp in astonishment. Last night a young man who is a guest here at the motel treated the desk clerk and me to an Italian dinner. It was delicious, and we had a good time. I'm getting anxious to get to Fort Myers, where I'll find a room and there is a college there—Edison Junior College. I have already been invited to a church there.

Once more I'll say, happy birthday, Grandpa, and I'll close with praise to God for the energy and guidance he has provided me (Divine Providence). God bless you and Grandma, too.

Love,
Sylvia

PS, I've already crossed one beautiful swamp (seventy-five miles), the Okefenokee Swamp in southern Georgia. The road was smooth and lined with water lilies, wildflowers, frogs, and tall, slender Australian pines. Those pines echoed back to me, *click, click, click, click* ...

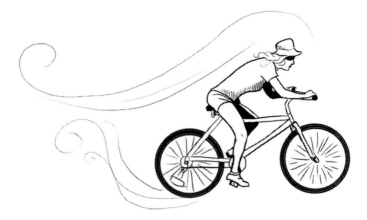

Song lyrics from my heart and *Song of the South*, Disney
Zippidy-do-da, zippidy ay,
My-o-my what a wonderful day.
Plenty of sunshine headin' my way—
Zippidy-do-daaa, zippidy-ay.

Mr. Bluebird on my shoulder
It's the truth, it's actual,
Everything is satisfactual.
Zippidy-do-da, zippidy ay,
Wonderful feelin', wonderful day.

Grandpa, the next trip is to Butte, Montana—shall we go together?

Grandpa Allen had been to Butte as a young man and dreamed of just hopping a freight car and going again.

I made it to Fort Lauderdale by August 26 and checked into a Howard Johnson Motel. A man stood next to me as I checked in with the young female desk clerk. When I completed the check-in process, the man invited both the clerk and me to have spaghetti with him at a local Italian restaurant. It was delightful company that evening. Before we got up from the table, the young man, who was a Cessna airplane dealer, invited me and my bicycle,

Jesse, to fly over the Everglades the next day. I hesitated but then agreed. However, it was not supposed to be.

The next morning I did another of my early-morning risings. I thought to myself, *I have to do this my way.* It was 4:30 a.m., so I left a note on the kind gentleman's door thanking him but telling him I had to finish my journey as intended, on bicycle. It was still pitch-dark outside and there was a chill in the air. I stopped for a quick breakfast at a diner and began making my way by the tiny light on my bicycle. Then something happened that I prayed was not an omen for the day—my light flashed onto something big by the side of the road. I stopped, backed up, and shone the light on it. Here, it was a dead cow lying there! I gasped and quickened my pace westward, away from the slightly sunlit eastern horizon.

My next obstacle was not so big, nor was it as ominous. I came to a toll booth at the entrance to Alligator Ally. I stood and studied the situation for a moment. It was getting light enough that I could see guard rails, maybe a foot and a half high, behind the booths. I resolutely walked my bicycle up to the rail, lifted it over, and then stepped over myself. I went riding down that two-lane road. As I did, the toll booth attendant came out, waving frantically, shouting, "Lady, you can't do that." I continued without hesitation but thinking to myself, *Well, you just watch me.*

Even though I talked big to my family because I wanted them to be proud of me—"I'm going to finish nursing school, get my license, and then even a bachelor's degree. I'm going to make it really big, folks!"—deep down all I wanted was to get to Naples. I felt like there was still a piece of me there. The day unfolding before me now was probably one of the most awesome parts of the journey—Alligator Alley. The sun rose behind me, and I saw wildlife scatter from the road ahead. The road's surface had a glow about it as the sunlight reflected from the asphalt, almost like a stream of water in front of me. At one point I decided to climb a fire tower to get a better view, but to do so, I had to climb an eight-foot chain-link fence, managing even to make it over the barbed wire at the top. A few scratches were little to pay for the bigger view from the tower.

At that hour there was little other traffic. I wondered if I might actually see an alligator. I was once again on my bicycle and making it further into the glades when I saw something quite long stretched out across the road, maybe a hundred feet in the distance. I thought to myself, *Oh, is it an alligator?* It frightened me at first, but the closer I got I realized it was only an old truck tire tread. I felt relieved but also a little disappointed.

By noon I found myself resting on my blanket at a rest stop. As I lay gazing up at the clear blue sky, an airplane seemed to be circling the area. Was it my friend the Cessna airplane salesman? I smiled as I waved, *"Thank you."* Alligator Alley was seventy-five miles long and known for its frequent thunderstorms over the Everglades. Storm-wise, the afternoon posed more threat. I saw huge thunderclouds forming above, and lightning lit up the sky in front of me. I pedaled frantically westbound, deluged by clouds bursting over me, drenching my head. The rainwater trickling over my sweaty skin tasted salty. The words of "Climb Every Mountain" from the movie Sound of Music rang through my head, "When you walk through a storm keep your head up high … and don't be afraid of the dark …" I recalled my father's reassuring words too, "Rubber tires on a vehicle keep it from being struck by lightning." I repeated over and over to myself, *You are okay, Sylvia, you are okay … You are okay, Sylvia, you are okay …* so many times, I actually felt okay. Besides, where I was coming from, my *City of Destruction*, was a great deal more frightening than any of this marvelous journey. I went on, reassuring myself over and over. Still, I was alone and vulnerable.

This aloneness, this time of precious introspection, meant so much to me. I felt like the Pilgrims once did. I had Divine Providence on my side. This was a time for me to examine and re-examine my values. I truly believed in only what was real, and people and animals, even vegetation, were real. I decided the best way to make up my mind as to what to do when two or more alternatives were given to me was to only act on what affected a living being! For example, if I were faced with free time and I could either work on a sewing project or go to see a friend in need of cheering and encouragement, the latter would be my choice because that living, breathing person takes precedence over an inanimate needle, spool of thread, and fabric. Or say I had a given amount of money saved in my bank account and I wanted to buy a new part for my bike with that money. Then I met a young woman on the street with a torn and tattered coat. Well, forget the bike part—that woman's needs would come first.

Throughout the trip I was bothered by thoughts of Sam—this man I barely knew but for the feel of his body. He was locked up in a penitentiary and at the mercy of the state of Florida and the judgments of so many people of greater authority. There was so much I did not understand about myself and how I got so involved with this strange but tender being. I could not effectively draw a line between real love and physical passion. How could I have had such ill-conceived notions to think a relationship would last between Sam and me? Where had it all come from? I dreaded to think where it might have taken me. My God, what if I had become pregnant with him—then what would I have done? I didn't become pregnant, but I still felt attached at the heart to him. I still loved him with a kind of innocent, simple love. I felt as young, or younger, than dear Pancake, the woman I met in jail. My thinking was, indeed, as simple as was hers.

> *Wheel going around and around, clicking, spinning, driving me further into life, away from, toward. Where have I begun, where have I been, where am I going? I just keep pedaling, around and around ... I saw what I saw, I see what I see, I will see what there is to see. Oh, wheel going around and around, clicking, spinning, driving me further, further, further ... When I stop, nobody knows; where I stop I know not either. I just am, I just am, I ... just ... am. I ... am ... I am ... I ... I ... I ... am ... am ... am ...*

Click, click, click, click ... water droplets ran from my hair into my eyes. I had to just keep going, not looking at my watch for the time nor at my odometer for distance. My mind was focused totally on the destination. Then I saw it, a sign with these blessed words: Naples—three miles. At 3:30 in the afternoon, I breezed into East Naples, my skin as dark as the inner husk of a coconut and seat as sore and red as an Amarillo blossom. I stopped a moment to breathe a prayer of thanksgiving and a sigh of absolute relief.

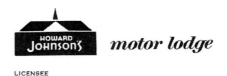

Saturday evening, August 26, 1972

Dear Family,

'tis a rugged road, more so than it seems,
To follow a pace so rambling and uncertain as that of the soul:
To penetrate the dark profundities of its intricate internal windings;
To choose and to lay hold of so many motions.

—Montaigne

The above quote is from an article by Peter Chew, "Everybody Is Lonely," *The National Observer*, August 12, 1972. It says a lot to me.

Today is a rainy day in Naples, a good day to rest and to go searching through the Collier County Library. I've hung up my pedals and taken to more stationary matters—those concerning food, clothing, and shelter. It's time to grow.

As I visited the library this morning I took out a book entitled *Pilgrim's Progress*, a Christian allegory written by John Bunyan. Christian is on a long journey from the City of Destruction to find the golden gate of the Lord's city, Zion. It is a strange though relevant story. The main character, Christian, travels through the "Slough of Despondency," the "City of Morality," "Fort Beelzebub," "Destruction," "The Valley of the Shadow of Death," "The Delectable Mountains," "Conceit," and "The Enchanted Ground" until he reaches his destination. Strangely enough, I feel I have passed through all these places. My morality has been tried, I've shaken hands with Beelzebub, and I've been captive in the Slough of Despondency. I have passed through the valley of the shadow of death several times. Now I believe I am at the delectable mountains, where the road is very clear. I can see my error. I am far from the journey's end, but hope is driving me on.

Really, you have to read the story to know what I am talking about. I'm so glad the Lord has seen me through this journey and safely to this place. I tried to make it to Fort Myers, as originally intended; however, circumstances told me this is not where I am to be. On the way I was nearly run over twice, and I was drenched by a half hour of solid downpour. This is more trouble than I had over the entire thousand miles.

So, here I am again in Naples. Father, I am using your credit for seven nights of rest, which I need to get ready to go job hunting this coming Monday. There are several good prospects. Tomorrow I move to a more-permanent residence, Rest Haven Motel, a small, older, and more homelike place on Eighth Avenue and within three blocks of downtown Naples. The people who own the place are in Connecticut, but the caretaker is a widow who has single handedly maintained all ten rooms, the grounds, and the finances. Ida Moore is her name, and she wants me to go to the beach with her tomorrow. I think she'll be good company.

My new acquaintances so far have been absolutely delightful. Mostly everyone wants to hear about my travels, although the subject is getting a bit tiring to me right now. Several young gentlemen acquaintances have required a good deal of reserve on my part. One gentleman, an airplane salesman from Kansas, offered—or shall I say insisted—on flying me from Fort Lauderdale over Alligator Alley to Fort Myers. However, that would have taken the satisfaction out of arriving at my destination, so I started out at 4:00 a.m. Wednesday morning. By noon I was halfway across the Alley. And as I lay resting at a traffic pull-off point by the side of the road, a huge "bird" flew overhead. It was him, I'm convinced, checking up on my progress.

Of my entire pilgrimage, this journey across Alligator Alley was the most beautiful. The sun rose behind me, clouds billowed high above me in a deep, blue, tropical sky, and miles and miles of visible road stretched out before me. Dozens of rabbits, birds, and tiny wild animals scurried off to the side of the road. I saw a red-headed woodpecker, dozens of large black vultures, a big, *big* owl (with "who, who, who" coming from it), and an alligator five feet long, which turned out to be a truck tire tread! At one place I hopped over a barbed-wire fence and climbed a fire tower. What a beautiful view and breeze. It took seven hours to cross the seventy-eight-mile stretch. At the end I was greeted by a very, very angry tollhouse attendant. Then the traffic commissioner came out of the nearby station: "How the *#!*#!!! did you get across there?" What a pleasant greeting for a tired pilgrim.

Oh, well, I'm here now. Thank you, God, for the energy and incentive to make it this far. As I said before, it is time to stop pedaling and start growing. Now the journey is inward, where the greatest treasures are stored. God bless my wonderful family. I hope and pray that you are all well.

Love,
Sylvia

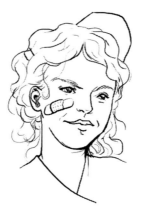

CHAPTER 3

Spinning

Wheel going around and around, clicking, spinning, driving me further into life, away from, toward. Where have I begun, where have I been, where am I going? I just keep pedaling, around and around … I saw what I saw, I see what I see, I will see what there is to see. Oh, wheel going around and around, clicking, spinning, driving me further, further, further … When I stop, nobody knows; where I stop I know not either. I just am, I just am, I … just … am. I … am … I am … I … I … I … am … am … am …

Yes, where am I going? It felt like I was spinning my *wheel* and getting nowhere, fast. I got a job again at that nice community hospital, but at seventy-five cents an hour! I remember thinking to myself, *Gee, can they afford me?* It felt almost like I was going backward instead of forward. And the cost of living in Naples was so high I prayed for a broom closet to live in; I certainly could not afford an apartment. I spent the next five years of my free time meandering by bicycle, *click, click, click, click,* through all the upper-class neighborhoods of Naples. I would work my tail off at the hospital—to the point of delirium—and come home with so much chest pain and spasms it was all I could do to sleep it off or to sleep at all for that matter.

At first I worked on the surgical unit at the hospital, giving the usual baths and back rubs, checking vital signs, post operative drainage, and dressings. I liked best of all to minister to the patients mindfully, giving them every encouragement I could. I would "talk them up," you might say. Then I was transferred to the medical unit upstairs, where the work got a great deal more involved—more running, more lifting, more everything. Mrs. Purslow was the head nurse, but I mostly worked under Mrs. Hill.

Most of us called Mrs. Hill by her first name, Angie. Angela Crismale Hill is what she kiddingly liked to call herself, and she was from New Jersey. Work was intense at the desk—the center of operation for that unit—and I appreciated Angie for her way of letting go. When things got too intense, she would retreat to the conference room behind the desk for a drag on her cigarette. Then we heard her say, "What am I, who am I, and what am I doing?" She would sigh, and I could see her whole body relax. Boy, she was good.

When I had a day or two off, I would come back to work feeling pretty good. But after only an hour or two of work, the spasms and chest pain would start all over. For a time I lived only three blocks from the hospital, but later I lived all the way up in North Naples at the Shady Rest Mobile Home Park. To get home, I usually rode all the way up Gulf Shore Boulevard, as far as I could, until I had to cut inland for home. That ride revived me. I chuckled a bit, going past fancy homes where the sprinkler systems clicked on at night, some of them broken and sending water over the road. Sweet jasmine bloomed over a split-rail fence, where the streetlight overhead illuminated its glorious yellow splendor. I would get home at 1:00 or 2:00 a.m. feeling revived, whip up a serving of hot pancakes with syrup, and then sink into a night of bizarre dreams.

DREAM, DREAM, DREAM ...

I am a twenty-six-year-old woman caught in an ongoing nightmare. I am lying in bed. I have learned how to put myself to sleep at night. I close my eyes to a dream of death. I imagine myself lying in a hospital bed, just like I did years ago as a child. I deeply desire to be in a place where I can freely say, "I hurt," And someone would respond and go for help. The good doctor would come into the room and say, "Sylvia, you are dying. There is nothing we can do." I feel the love of my family around me.

I drift into a disturbed sleep. *I am dying. There is nothing anyone can do.*

Going to work was challenging in that I felt so bad from the pain, I had to work up the adrenalin to get going again. This often took an hour, maybe two. Then I became super nurse and would hurt myself all over, doing things I know today I had no business doing. But in 1972, I was in so much denial I could not stop the progression of this insane behavior. I did not even know what it was that made me so miserable from working. It was just annoying *feelings*. Had I known the origin, I could have told Dr. Ricketts, whose office I frequented, and maybe he could have talked some sense into me. He could have told me how much damage I was doing myself. Instead, all he could do was bring in a big ol' hypodermic full of a red solution I knew to be Vitamin B12.

After that first week staying in a tiny little motel room, paid for by my father again, I found a room on North Third Street. It was a lovely room off the breezeway of a retired couple's home. I had no kitchen or even a refrigerator. I frequented a restaurant called The Clock down near the bend in the Tamiami Trail, where the road turned eastward. One little red-headed waitress with a little boy at home became my friend and confidante. When I ran out of money, which I frequently did, I ate leftovers off the patients' trays at work. I never ate so much egg custard in my life! At one point I wanted to get ahead financially and took on a second job at Lums, a pizza restaurant.

Tuesday, September 5, 1972

Dear Grandma,

I am sitting in a Laundromat with my feet propped up on a chair and my sneakers in the washer. The sun is shining, and I am thinking of you. Are you okay? Happy birthday. This is my day off from the hospital, and tomorrow too. I really need it, as I worked seven straight nights from four in the afternoon to twelve and one o'clock in the morning for Lum's, an eating place here. However, last night was my last night at the restaurant, because I want to give all my time and energy to my hospital work. However, I was glad for the extra work in order to get my expenses paid in advance.

It is expensive living here in Naples, Florida, but it is worth it to have the privilege of working with these nurses. They are excellent examples of what a really professional person can be. And when I come back [to Harrisburg], I hope to bring that example to my hometown. The Polyclinic Hospital and school, in particular, are in need of stamina and a newfound incentive. [I must have been speaking more for myself here.]

Grandma, are the tomatoes full and heavy on the vines? The lady who keeps the motel where I stayed last week brought some tomatoes along on the picnic this past Sunday. Most of the tomatoes down here, according to her, are a bit, I believe you would call them, pithy. And they were. Our picnic was in Seminole Indian State Park. Both of us were wearing bright green dresses and sunglasses. Mrs. Moore, the motel keeper and a very respectable friend, has pure blond-white hair. She's a very lovely person. We sat at a picnic table beneath some palm trees.

I wish you and Grandpa could see how beautiful it is here. There is at least one drenching rainstorm every day, and then the sun comes out bright.

Mrs. Moore and I went to the First Presbyterian Church. The singing and parable lesson made me cry. It was a real joy.

God bless you, Grandma.

Love,
Sylvia

PS Please tell Grandpa I got his nice little note.

I am grateful Mother kept quite a number of my letters home. For one thing, they reflect the kind of moralizing and fundamentalism that went on in my overworked, confused brain. Being the child of business-minded folks, we were always dubbing this person *good*, or that person *not so good*, referring, of course, more to their work ethics than their personalities. Still, many of my letters were in judgment of others, especially when it came to their behavior around the opposite sex. Whether they were living together before marriage was a big one in my book of "no-nos." My Grandmother and Grandfather Allen especially had this influence on me. Grandmother had been raised Brethren, and she was not allowed to even dance. Personally, I don't know how I could have gone without dancing, because of that part of me akin to a Mexican jumping bean.

I was so simple minded, and I was only just beginning to put my life and my thinking together. It was much like Christian meeting *Mr. Worldly Wiseman* on the road to the *Celestial City*. I was on a tangent, a side road, looking to meet *Mr. Legality* and his son, *Civility*, in the town of *Morality*. I felt so vulnerable, but these thoughts must have somehow been empowering to me. I was alone and feeling lost.

Here is one letter that reflects the judgmental mentality going on in my head:

Friday October 6, 1972

Dear Father, ♪

This is just a little note to say I love you. Are you okay? [This was a time in his life when his heart was really starting to fail him, and he had such a desire to live.] I miss you, but I am happy. My days end with such satisfaction—especially today.

Last evening I had a young man come visit me. He had been a patient of mine at the community hospital, and I invited him to come visit me at the Benders'. So he came and

95

we talked and listened to radio [on the porch outside my room] for about three hours. He knew I was here in Naples by myself, and I sensed that he was rather underhandedly questioning my principles in life. For example, he asked, "Do you believe in the new generation ... and, like, living together without being married?"

After he left, I found myself deep in thought. Questions, questions, questions—is it for us, the "new generation" to change the standards that have been given to us by our Christian forefathers? After all, I am part of this generation, whether I conform to their behavior or not.

I am especially satisfied at the end of this day because I feel strong. I've asked questions of my peers and my patients. My belief is upheld. One patient, a blind, decrepit old lady of about eighty years of age, even supplied me with the affection that only a Christian heart could supply. Now I am happy and ready to answer to the young man's questions more firmly. I know by the manner in which he conducts himself that he respects me. However, his conversation has not been very enlightening, so he has only one more chance. We're going to dinner tomorrow night.

I called Tom Chadwick at Southern Motors [the Renault dealership] in Savannah, Georgia, yesterday to tell him I would be arriving Saturday morning if someone would be there to give me my car and belongings. Unfortunately, he goes out of town on weekends, so I've requested two consecutive weekdays off next week, Thursday and Friday, to make the trip. I should be able to do it in one day, but it would be good to have a day to rest before returning to work.

Father, would you believe, one of my patients—a fellow about twenty-eight years of age—was admitted to the hospital as an attempted suicide because he walked off the end of the pier? But in a brief conversation with him, I found out his true motive was not suicide. He thought he was God and was trying to walk on water! It is difficult to bring a person like this back to reality and to recognize his own identity. I attempted to do this by questioning him as to his state of being mortal. I took his blood pressure and pulse and then said very discretely, "You're the same as me or the patient here next to you—a physical being. You are growing old like the rest of us!" He acknowledged this without controversy. This was good.

I wonder how a man could develop such a false identity or self-image, so I inquired as to his home life. "Oh, I've been traveling for two years or more," he replied. "I have no home." I thought to myself, *This is how he got this way. He had not stopped long enough to find himself or to let his own heart and mind be tried by the people in any one place. People are the only true reflection of their own souls.* Don't you agree? I think you do, because you are my father and I love you. God bless you.

Love,
Sylvia

PS. At choir Wednesday night we sang a Scottish Christmas carol with a high descant and the basses singing, "Bam, bam, bam," like drummers. We sang in the sanctuary of First Presbyterian Church. It was beautiful. Did you know Paul said in Philippians 4:9–11, "Those things, which ye have both learned and received, and heard and seen in me do, and the God of peace shall be with you. Not that I speak in respect of want: for I have learned in whatsoever state I am, therewith to be content."

Being tired →rest
Being hungry →seek food
Being lonely →seek fellowship
Being put off →take time to reconsider
Being neglected →take refuge in the Lord

By October I was able to retrieve my car. Leave it to my father and his good sense. He had it towed to Savannah, where a Renault dealership repaired it for thirty-five dollars. Had I left Bozo in Orangeburg repair it, I would have been a real sucker. It was nice to have the car back, but it did not feel like me anymore to be driving. By now Sam had also already been transferred to a prison work camp just outside Naples. I felt remotely attached to him, enough that by his birthday in November, I got permission to bring a picnic lunch and take him out. Oh my, such foolishness.

I no sooner picked Sam up and the old behaviors began again. There were plenty of picnic spots along the Trail, but we rolled past all of them and ended up out of Sam's legal limit—Fort Myers! I found myself once again sitting on a bar stool ordering screwdrivers, intoxicated to the tipping point. I knew I had to get him back. We were rolling in the right direction, at least, when Sam said to me, "Pull over, Sylvia." Not knowing what he had in mind, I pulled over. He bolted from the car. That was the last I saw of him.

A week later I got a phone call from North Carolina. It was Sam. "Sylvia," I heard a muffled voice say on the other end, "I'm desperate. Can you wire me some money to a Western Union here?"

By now realizing what a taker this young man was, I replied, "Yeah, Sam, I'll send you some money." But inside I knew what I had to do. I called the Collier County Sherriff's Department and told them where Sam was, waiting for my supposed money transfer. They no doubt picked him up, because two days later, his mother, Mrs. McQueen called me, ranting and raving over the phone about what a lousy person I was. It was an easy hang up on my end; it was over.

By January I was not only burning out royally from work, with the kind of pain I lived with and the demanding pace of work, but I was also starting to feel pretty lonely. Not only was I miserable from pain, but I was also getting sick from the flu that was going around. I had the weekend off and nobody in particular to spend it with. The retired army captain and his wife where I lived treated me more like an ill-begotten stray than a tenant. That was okay; they were kind of ol' fogies anyway. So I gravitated to a bar and lounge again that was off the south end of the trail. It just felt good to be around people. I sat staring into a margarita, my thoughts drifting to the sound of a lady tickling the keys of the piano while singing "Autumn Leaves." Inevitably, I met someone.

This time it was a tall, thin sort of fellow in his thirties. Tommy was a retired navy marine mechanic. We made it back to my room by the wee hours of the morning. Now I knew I was not supposed to have men in my quarters, but my fever was raging. I was too sick to care about any rules. I had at least the wherewithal to insist the door to the breezeway be left open. I hoped it would dispel any sense of hanky-panky going on it that little room. Tommy just sat by my bedside all night, giving me water, reassuring me. It was nice to be cared for, for a change. Regardless, that morning the captain came out and threw us both out. I tried to explain, "I've been so sick, Captain, and Tommy just sat with me." But the rules were the rules, unmerciful as they seemed, and I was out of there!

I had nowhere else to go, so wouldn't you guess? I ended up living on a small cabin cruiser with Tommy on the city dock to the Gordan River. Boy, did we rock that boat too that first couple of weeks. When the city restricted living off the dock, Tommy found a houseboat moored at the Cove Inn. We could live there while he worked on it, but first he had to bring it up off the bottom of the river. My job was to help clean it up on the inside. On my hours off from the hospital, I found myself shoveling muck. I will never forget that first night.

We were asleep in a cubby on the upper part of the boat. The chandeliers from the inn dining room just across the way gave our little houseboat some soft light, and there was a party going on in the boat next to us. It was pleasant hearing soft conversation and laughter, with the music made by ice cubes in drinking glasses. That night, after an evening of hard drinking together, I dreamed that we were sinking and warm water was coming up beneath me. I awoke suddenly, only to realize Tommy had pissed the bed. I was some disgusted at this. But thus far he had been nothing but kind to me. Unlike Sam, he was mature and definitely more responsible. One evening, once the houseboat was up off the river bottom, we sat eating a bushel of raw oysters off the stern. Interestingly, the boat was named *Walking and Talking*.

And we did; we talked and talked. We had both been lonely, but I could not help feeling Tommy was wounded as well. He had come to Naples from North Carolina, leaving his two daughters with their grandparents. I asked what happened to his wife. He responded, "She committed suicide."

This little shocking bit of information startled me, but it softened my heart toward him even more. I did not ask the details, but I could read the sadness in his eyes.

Collier County had a technical school, and a new program to train practical nurses was in its pilot stage. The first class of nurses had begun in January. One of the instructors, a Mrs. Munroe, had seen me at work many times. She saw I was skilled in nursing, so she approached me one day. "Sylvia, why don't you join our nursing class?"

By now it was March of 1973, and I would have to get caught up to the other students. Not a problem—Polyclinic was a sound medical-surgical background. For the next nine months, I donned my little pin-striped blue uniform with the white Peter Pan collar and became, once again, a student nurse. It was the story of my life!

Within the month, Tommy and I were forced to move again. This time we took our "house" with us. *Walking and Talking* was towed further inland to a canal marina, where Tommy could work on it with the benefit of a shop and tool shed. I sold the car, so I was back to pedaling everywhere, the way I liked it. I was able to cut my work hours for the time being to have study time. I felt very little passion toward this new guy in my life compared to the raging passion Sam and I had shared. Tommy was just a man, someone I could lean on, someone for whom I could prepare a meal, watch him shovel it in, and then linger over the empty plates. I wanted him to talk more about his past, but everything stopped cold with his wife's suicide.

By April I was growing accustomed to this new life. Tommy worked hard at the marina. Not much was done on our houseboat, however. He worked on a number of other boats, the biggest challenge being to revive the motors. Of course a marina is not exactly considered a residential area. We were more like squatters, with no taxes, no listing in the phonebook, and no ordinary services like paper delivery or garbage pickup. One Sunday afternoon a call came into the office. It was for me. I heard my father's voice on the other end, "Sylvia, we've not heard from you. Are you doing okay?"

"Oh, hi, Father. Why, yes, I'm doing just dandy. I am living on a houseboat at a marina, and my *friend* Tommy's been looking after me. We're both fine."

There was an awkward moment of silence on the other end until he replied, "Should we be getting to know this young fellow? I mean, have you two made any commitments? I can only assume you are living together."

I wanted to ask, "What business is it of yours? I'm a grown woman." But I didn't. Mother and Father had put up with so much with me. I knew they did not condone living together before marriage. Then I filled him in as to how school was going and my work, never mentioning what I felt from day to day. Feelings had simply never been the center of any of our conversations that I could remember. Besides, to what end would it come telling him how physically miserable I was?

After about ten minutes more of saying sweet nothings, we finally hung up. The whole conversation must have stimulated a bout of guilt in me, because the very next day I went to my minister, Pastor Stump, at First Presbyterian Church and asked if he would perform a wedding ceremony for Tommy and me. Fortunately, the pastor knew just the right questions to reinforce the fact that I knew so little of this man I was living with.

"Are you sure this is the man you want to spend the rest of your life with?" he asked.

May and then June were upon us. I was making my daily weekday trek by bicycle to the hospital and then home. I only had until January to complete the nursing course. Being more inland, we did not have the usual off-shore breezes at the marina. I liked to swim in the canal to cool off and relax. The water was murky, and one day I had a visitor. A big, rounded creature swam by me, startling me. The marina owner, Carl, heard me scream and saw me swim frantically for the boat. He explained I was in the company of a sea cow or manatee. He reassured me, "She won't bother you if you don't bother her." Still, the canal suddenly seemed too small for us both.

Fishermen came and went out of the marina, and we were often the partakers of the extras from a big catch. One night I cleaned and fried some trout. Tommy enjoyed having me cook for him, naturally. When we were done, I wrapped the remains in old newspaper and threw it in an open barrel right outside Tommy's shop. On the afternoon of the next day, I rode in from work. Tommy was struggling with a motor, a stubborn one he had been trying for weeks to get running. As I greeted him and approached him with a smile, my lips puckered for a kiss, I failed to realize that he had had to work all day with the stench of decaying fish remains right next to him. I noticed, however, that *something* was wrong. The grey eyes that had been deep and loving were now sending shards of glass and bolts of lightning, cutting me. What was wrong? I saw him raise his arm, but before he could bring it down on me, I ducked out the door.

That night I slept restlessly, and Tommy was out until 2:00 a.m. In the morning I awoke to a disturbing dream. In the dream I saw him standing before me, but instead of a head and upper torso, he was a baseball bat. Then I knew this is why Tommy's wife committed suicide. I was not going to stick around to find out anymore. No need to—*S*pirit had fed me who Tommy really was; he was an abuser.

The next day I shared my desperate need to find other living arrangements with a fellow student, Paulette. That evening she helped me move into her home temporarily. This was a kind gesture because her husband was not very keen on my presence. Feeling homeless and desperate, it was difficult, to say the least. Then add work, school, and continuous physical pain and what was left but a torn, miserable young lady? The wisdom of leaving Tommy was even more apparent when I went back to retrieve the last of my things. In a fit of anger, Tommy had kicked the floor fan all the way to the other side of the cabin, where it lay in a dozen or more pieces. Good God that could have been me!

I was growing weary of this town full of snowbirds and retirees. I didn't mind bald heads—in fact I found them appealing—but I needed young people around me. One person, perhaps a little older than me, was a lab technician named Anna. I saw her frequently at work in the hospital. She would come into a lot of the rooms where I was working to draw blood from the patients.

During a conversation with Anna, I revealed my need for better living arrangements. Anna was a tall, slender and very gentle young woman. She told me she lived in the hospital apartments. I thought to myself, *Well, I'm a hospital worker. Why shouldn't I have an apartment there too?*

"Anna," I said, "would you like a roommate?"

She hesitated, deep in thought. Then I heard her quiet voice say, "I wouldn't mind." I felt my heart leap. Well, now, this would surely be my broom closet—probably better.

Anna had a one-bedroom apartment with twin beds, a large living room, and a kitchen-dinette area. I think it felt a little awkward to us both. For me it was quite livable. It bothered me a little that she was so quiet. I wished she would share just a little of herself. One morning in particular really got on my nerves.

One of her coworkers had a birthday, and Anna decided to make a coconut cake for her, the hard way. Early that morning, I heard her out there whipping up this cake from scratch. She even split a whole coconut and ground the white flesh to a fine consistency. There was so much banging around I was afraid to even go out. On her way out, she even managed to slam the back door so hard I thought surely Anna was angry with me. I went out to find the kitchen in a sad state of disarray. It wasn't my mess, but being a bit obsessive, I went about cleaning it up as best I could.

As with many girl-girl dwelling arrangements, one sooner or later finds a beau. In fact, I wondered if having a roommate did not encourage Anna to move on. God knows. He no doubt had a plan for Anna, because before long I saw a glimmer in her eyes that told me one thing.

I asked, "Anna, you have a boyfriend don't you?" The question seemed to open a floodgate between Anna and myself.

"Yes, I have, Sylvia, and his name is Charlie. I met him at church. He's coming by. Would you like to meet him?"

"Of course, Anna, I would love to."

Anna and Charlie were both born-again, devout Christians. I suspect my being in the apartment delayed some of the intimacy they might have had were I not there. And this may have, in a way, helped them. Still, I soon started to feel like a fifth wheel, like, *"Get lost, roomie."* They were both too kind to just push me out, but I got the message.

So I did what I always did. I went home hunting again. This time I rode my little blue Raleigh bike up North Tamiami Trail. I hoped as I got further out of town I would find cheaper but private living arrangements. Everything in town was out of my price range. About three miles out, I came upon a mobile home court. A small, dual-axel, green trailer sat two lots in from the trail. A sweet, slightly stooped little grey-haired woman was shaking a carpet out. I approached with my friendly, "Hello."

"Why, hello," she responded "Won't you come in? I just made a pot of homemade potato soup."

I leaned my bicycle against a coconut palm and went in. The aroma of the soup filled that whole little nineteen-foot camper, making my mouth water. It was a tiny little place. Her husband was sitting on the couch watching the news on an eighteen-inch television screen. The smell of that delicious soup and their friendliness made it feel like a palace inside. The couple, from Ohio, was hungry for any morsel of information I could give them about myself. After telling them the story of my escape from the *City of Destruction*, I finally shared with them my need for a place to live. I saw the woman's eyebrows go up. "Why, we could use someone to inhabit our camper here while we go back up north for the summer." Small wonder.

Several days later, Charlie and Anna were kind enough to help me move once again. By now they were planning a March 17 wedding, and they wanted me to sing for it. Anna went to her home in Bushnell at the beginning of the week while Charlie and I were to come up that Friday. Charlie could get my goat at times. He would kid around and talk from his butthole. He was entertaining but annoying too at times. He reminded me, disgustingly, of my brother up in Pennsylvania. But he was a likeable, sensitive young man; so I was happy for Anna.

The Friday before the wedding Charlie picked me up to travel up and to inland Florida. He had a little cabin cruiser boat attached to the rear of his green Pontiac sedan. Soon we were heading up the trail, Charlie's mouth going a thousand words a minute. The more he spoke, the sillier he got, until he started to play with the steering wheel. The car swerved, and next thing you know, the bow of the boat behind us picked the rear end of the car up off the road! God must have been with us, because instead of throwing our vehicle off the road, the boat became detached and rolled across the opposing lane and into a ditch.

Whew. We sat silent a moment, collecting ourselves, thanking God no cars had been coming in the opposite direction. Then, without another word, he turned the car around and we went back for the boat, reattached it, and once again made our way north. A mile further we came upon a roadside drive-in movie marquee advertizing, *Charlie's Angels*. Only then did Charlie speak, "That *had* to be the work of angels back there." I sighed and said under my breath, "I hope they're still watching."

*Wheel going around and around, clicking, spinning, driving
me further into life, away from, toward. Where have I
begun, where have I been, where am I going? I just keep
pedaling, around and around … I saw what I saw, I see
what I see, I will see what there is to see. Oh, wheel going
around and around, clicking, spinning, driving me further,
further, further … When I stop, nobody knows; where I
stop I know not either. I just am, I just am, I … just … am.
I … am … I am … I … I … I … am … am … am …*

My new place, the little travel trailer, was one of the coziest I had ever
lived in. It was, realistically, my broom closet. There was no air conditioning
either. Wow could that place get warm during the summer. Two lots up
and toward the center of the park there was an eighty-five-year-old widower
named Gus. He was a really lonely old guy. When I had a free morning, I
would go over just to visit. Several times he invited me over for beer, cheese,
and crackers. When it came time to leave I'd say, "Gus, I gotta go now."
Invariably, he would reach to turn up the hearing aid in his shirt pocket
and say, "What did you say? I can't hear you." We would have a chuckle
together. I sensed he was getting pretty attached to me. He was a kind and
gentle man.

I was glad to be where I was because good friends of mine from church
choir, big, tall Bill Hemmer, a truancy officer for the schools, and his lovely,
petite wife, Marjorie, lived only a mile up the road. One day I was on my
way to visit them when I heard a desperate meow coming from a trench full
of weeds at the side of the road. It was a tabby, grey kitten, his fur matted
and covered with tar. He could not have been more than eight weeks old;
he was so tiny. I quickly snatched him up, took him home, and worked at
getting the tar off with turpentine and lots of good warm, soapy water. His
little green eyes and soft pink tongue stole my heart. I quickly named him
Tiger, like a similar cat I had growing up back in Harrisburg.

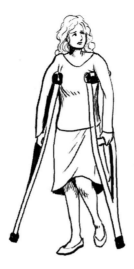

About this time, in April of 1974, I was finished with my nursing course. I had even passed the state licensing exam. It was April 14, and the days were still short. I was pretty much a loner by now. In fact, this particular day I was alone, except for my kitty, all day. I had been baking sugar cookies, and the camper still smelled sweet. The sun was just going down when suddenly the walls felt like they were coming in on me. I was having a panic attack, although at the time all I knew was the sheer terror. I left my kitty to play on the couch, grabbed a brown paper bag with some cookies, and took off on my bicycle for the Hemmers' home.

I got all the way there, and imagine that, they were not home. If only I had been able to call first. I turned around and headed back down the busy trail for home. By now it was getting dark. There was a bicycle path off to the side of the road, but most of it was covered with drifted sand. I had a light on my handlebars, plus two on the back, and I was riding frantically when suddenly I found myself flying through the air. The paper bag of cookies flew out of my hand, and I landed on the side of the road. The sand softened the landing, but when I tried to get up, I couldn't. Whoever hit me must have kept right on going. A little yellow Volkswagen beetle stopped just ahead, and a girl got out. Approaching me, she said, "Do you want a drink of my Coke?" I appreciated the offer, but right then I just needed help getting up.

It was not long until a police officer stopped and an ambulance came. I knew Jack, one of the EMTs. In fact, the year before I heard him say on the department at work, "That girl is going to get hit some day!" Well, thanks a lot, Jack, here I am, broken, just like you predicted. You were right, but I'm still not road kill. Except for getting a little shocky when they were taking x-rays at the hospital, I pulled out of it pretty quickly.

The next morning I found myself in a hospital bed on the fourth floor. I had a broken pubic bone and a huge contusion on the back of my left thigh, where the car headlight had hit me. One of my favorite nurse cohorts, Mrs. Thomas, came in to check on me. She stood at the end of the bed and said, "Sylvia, how are you doing this morning?" Now, there was no way I could have known what was going to happen next. Neither Mrs. Thomas nor I knew that the grapefruit I had eaten before the accident the night before was sitting like a time bomb in my stomach. Like a garbage disposal in reverse, the grapefruit hit the wall just behind where she was standing. I was so embarrassed. Mrs. Thomas, like any good nurse would do, just smiled and quietly went about getting the mess cleaned up.

About mid morning I got a call from my friend Anna's husband, Charlie. He had retrieved little Tiger to care for him until I got back home. About two minutes into the conversation, Charlie said, "Sylvia, I have to hang up a minute." The phone went dead. A few minutes later, he called me back. "Sylvia, I don't know how to tell you this, but your kitty was playing when he fell off my lap, landed on the concrete floor, and broke his neck! Sylvia, he's dead." I gasped. I heard Charlie's voice grow soft and apologetic. All I could think was, *I wonder what the stars said for me these last couple of days.*

Two days later I was discharged on crutches to go back to my little travel trailer. I was glad that over the last couple of years I had frequented a church, First Presbyterian Church, in town and sung in the choir. Yes, I was told I had a wonderful voice. One favorite old hymn I liked to sing was "His Eye Is on the Sparrow." The words, "Why should I feel discouraged, Why should the shadows come, Why should my heart be lonely ... And long for Heav'n and home ..." rang true to my heart. I was becoming all those things: discouraged and longing for home. I longed for intimacy and truly a place to call my own. I did not know where home was anymore. I did, however, feel someone was watching me through all this.

Don Ryno, the choir director and a marvelous organist, and his cohort, Seth, came to take me home from the hospital. They were two of my favorite men, and having them drive me home made me feel like royalty. For the next six weeks I hobbled around on crutches. Many of the choir members brought me casseroles. Ole Gus either cooked for me or took me to the grocery store. Going to the store with Gus proved to be a test of raw nerves. The Publix Grocery Store was only across North Tamiami Trail from our park. However, there was no signal to get us there, and traffic was heavy. Gus hollered, "Sylvia, hang on!" and floored it. That old silver-and-green, eight-cylinder Pontiac sped across the road, leaving a trail of rubber. I could feel the hair standing up on the back of my neck as I covered my eyes and scrunched down in the seat. Is what just happened what I think happened?

"Gus, were you trying to get us killed?" Gus did not answer; he had a way of not hearing when it did not suit him. Gus was really one of the nicest old guys, and I met a lot of retirees over the five years I was in Naples. Darn, if I had only been a few decades older, he would have made a marvelous helpmate. Why, he even ironed his sheets; I saw it with my own eyes.

So, there I sat, or tried to sit, in my tiny little trailer waiting for my six weeks of recovery to be over, each morning taking a few more steps without the crutches. One day I wanted so badly to see the Gulf that I took off on my crutches to try and walk the three miles to the beach. This was more foolishness on my part because I had to turn back when I got within a quarter mile of it. My armpits were sore and my shoulders ached from the crutches. That evening I got a call from home. Yes, I finally broke down and had a phone put in. I had to for the sake of my sanity. It was Mother, and she thought it might be a good idea for my sister, Wendy, to come spend time with me over the summer. My heart swelled with the thought of her coming. When I shared the news with Gus, he insisted on letting him take me to pick her up at the airport. I wanted to say, "But Gus, I want her to come stay with me, not die with me." However, I knew it would be all right. Surely my run of bad luck was over.

Naples, with all its charm, romantic appeal, and hard work, was really just an escape plan for me. Mostly it was an escape from Mother. This is awful to admit, but inside I vowed I would not go home until my mother was dead. Seeing Wendy get off that plane a week later made it feel a little like home was coming to me. Her hair was the usual light brown, medium length. She was so petite, and she still had the little monkey grin that always reminded us not to take life too seriously. Grandpa Gus was so sweet to us; he took us to dinner that night. The weather man was calling for a hurricane to be coming at us from the east, which meant we probably would not get the brunt of it, just the rain.

And we did. It rained for a solid week! To our horror, especially Wendy's, the lightning kept hitting the chain link fence at the dealership across the alley from us. The poor dear sat up every night for a week watching Betty Davis reruns on our little portable TV while I lay snoring in the back. That was not how I planned on entertaining her that week. As soon as the rain stopped, she rode my somewhat beat-up old Raleigh toward town, looking for work for the summer. It didn't take her long to get a job at Baskin Robins, selling ice cream, sundaes, and shakes. She regretted this after a while; the sampling was starting to show on her hips. However, bicycling back and forth helped keep her weight gain at a minimum.

I was so glad when June rolled around and I was able to throw my crutches over the handlebars of the bicycle and ride to the hospital, to return them and let them know in the nursing office I was ready for work. Also, it was getting awfully warm in our little camper—too warm for Wendy and not real suitable for the two of us. I went by my old room on North Third Street to find Mrs. Bender and the captain doing some yard work. I should have been a lawyer too, because before the conversation was over, I had convinced them to let me have my old room back. I think it had played on Mrs. Bender's guilt because I had been so sick on the day they threw me out. Now having Wendy here, things were different. I even found out they had put a refrigerator in the big walk-in closet. I was so glad to get back into town.

By now Wendy had only been with me a few weeks, and she was not real happy with her ice cream job, so she applied at the donut shop in town. I don't know if it was that discouraging first week with the lightning and the rain or if she just got homesick, but suddenly she wanted to go back to Pennsylvania. I tried not to show how heart sick I was when she took the bike the captain had loaned her and rode back to the donut shop to return her apron. But then something happened that made her decision seem like a wise one.

She had no sooner returned the apron and was crossing the Trail in front of the donut shop when a big Cadillac ran the red light and knocked her clean into the air. She came down on the guy's windshield and slid to the hot pavement. An African American man jumped from the vehicle, screaming, "Lordy, please don't let her be dead!" In an effort to escape the hot pavement, Wendy scrambled to her feet right away, but a nearby pedestrian insisted she lay back down—and cook—and wait for the ambulance. She tried to get up again. "The hospital is on the next block. I'll just walk." she said. Still no one would let her up, and she lay there frying like a couple of overcooked eggs. The next day she was on the plane flying back to Pennsylvania, taking a piece of my broken heart with her, but I understood.

Those first few years in Naples I pretty much romanticized it—the salty Gulf breezes, the coconut palms, the blue jays coming south in the winter, and the feeling I was making it on my own. But after my accident, things started to change. In addition to the chest pain and spasms in my face, now I was having problems in my lower torso. I had been back at work for close to two years by this time. And since I was a licensed nurse, they were actually paying me three dollars an hour! I honestly felt like I had it made, except for one thing: they were still working me to the bone. Not only that, but for reasons no one knew at the time, I was the least practical nurse in their employ.

There were definitely cogs missing in my head. I would have loved to have been assigned as a medication nurse, but the one time Angie put me on the med cart, I fouled up so badly I had a number of incident reports to write. I even put ear drops in a patient's eyes. Oh my, what a dunce. I knew better, but I just could not seem to get it right. I felt so frantic inside, hopeless.

I worked and I worked and I worked … Many a time I would look at Cheezie, short for Chessborough, the regular med nurse, and look at the other nurses and think to myself, *How do they do it?* I honestly thought they felt most of what I was feeling. In June of 1976, my friend Janet, who worked in the office of a general practitioner, Dr. Barnes, had gotten pregnant. She convinced him to hire me in her absence. I was elated, but I was also oppressed by those ominous symptoms I was having.

I kept going to Dr. Fox, the gynecologist, because I had pain in my pelvic area, possibly from it having been broken. Each time I went, he would say the same thing: "No, Sylvia, there is really nothing out of the ordinary down here."

Then, on my final visit to him, I lay on the exam table, feet in the stirrups. When he was just rolling his stool away from the exam table, I literally cried out, "Help me. Can't you please help me!" His brow furrowed to the frantic nature of my plea, as he told me, "Sylvia, you may be having back problems, and the pain is radiating from your spine. But just to be sure, I am going to admit you to the hospital to do a laparoscopy, where you will be put under anesthesia and a scope will be introduced at the umbilicus, or belly button, in order to examine the organs from a different perspective." Either way, I guess he figured a brief stay in the hospital couldn't hurt anything.

It was November of 1976 when I was admitted to the hospital for that laparoscopy. Dr. Fox came to my room after the procedure to report his findings. "Sylvia," he said, "your belly is so full of adhesions from the pelvis having been broken that I could not get the scope in far enough to see much of anything."

He also recommended seeing an orthopedic physician to look at my lower back. This would have been enough to satisfy me, but then he added, "I want the psychiatrist, Dr. Lombillo, to consult with you while you're here at the hospital too."

Now, from having worked on the third floor all those years I knew this psychiatrist to be overbooked to the hilt. How could one man possibly know so many people and be able to help them with the myriad of issues they surely presented to him? He was given consultations with everybody and their cousins. I was not too sure I wanted to be one of his subjects. What could he possibly know about my sense of suffering? He had surely not walked a day in my shoes. When he handed me a blank piece of paper on a clipboard and asked me to draw a man and a woman, I was sure he needed the consultation, not me. In an effort to make light of the whole thing, I drew an unorthodox picture: a man and a woman sitting nude on the beach.

Well, I can only guess this bizarre drawing got some unorthodox comments at the nurses' station. Even Dr. Barnes must have seen it, because the next day Janet came to my room and said to me in a compassionate voice, "Sylvia, Dr. Barnes has changed his mind and hired someone else for the office position."

Well, at least *I* got a good laugh from my artwork. Believe you me, though, it ended in tears. The mild depression that had been a way of life all those years suddenly turned to a deep chasm of despair. The day I was to be discharged, the director of nursing, Johanna, came to see me. I think she had been informed of my dire straits and simply wanted to encourage me somehow. She was pointing to my hometown. Slowly, a little light was beginning to flicker, showing me what I had to do.

When I got out of the hospital, I went to that orthopedic doctor, who took a whole barrage of x-rays. Nothing—absolutely nothing—showed. I also was checked out by an internist who also found, again, absolutely nothing. I was beginning to hit brick wall after brick wall, and with each hit, my morale dropped even lower. January of 1977 was the coldest winter I had spent in Naples. I remember looking out the window on the third floor at work and seeing snowflakes drift past. Was I still in southwest Florida? At the pier one day, I heard someone comment, "Who left the door to the north open?"

The cold was adding to my misery. Then one Wednesday my friend Anne, who sang with me in the church choir, came to have dinner with me before rehearsal. Still not having kitchen access, I used the hibachi grill out back. We had surf and turf or shrimp and pieces of juicy steak on shish kabobs. I pumped the gas on my little Coleman camper stove and cooked little red potatoes. At around 5:30, a gentle knock came on the wood frame of the outer screen door. Tall, gentle Anne stood with her hand over her brow, peering into the porch, which was lit softly by the evening sun. Soon we sat, butter dripping from our chins, soaking up delightful companionship. Just her being there was so precious. Then, to my greatest pleasure, Anne just started to talk. She and my other best friend, Joanne, were getting married within two months of each other. As for me, I was meeting absolutely no one—nada. It did not help at all that when I had time off I spent the whole time recovering from those *feelings*. There must be a God in heaven!

"Sylvia," she said, "you've been depressed, haven't you? I can tell."

I felt tears sting my eyes. She had hit it just right, because not only was I depressed, but the ache in my chest had mushroomed into a very, *very* lonely heart. Was there no one out there for me? Was there no way I could work and not be in constant pain? Even singing in the choir on Sunday mornings was a challenge for the simple reason that I often worked the night before and was in serious discomfort. By now I realized my tongue was stubbornly slipping to the right side of my mouth. On the days when I was overly tired, it was even hard to speak, much less sing. Now I had this wonderful friend here, just for me, and she seemed to have some insight into my life.

I nodded yes to her question. I was indeed getting more depressed with each passing day. She continued, "Sylvia, I have been praying about you. I really believe if you go back to your hometown in Pennsylvania, you will meet your husband there."

I could not believe what I was hearing. Could she be right? If she was, that meant someone could be waiting there for me right then! This was something I wanted more than anything. All the big talk about going back to school to get my RN and then maybe getting a bachelor's degree—well, that is all it was, talk. Inside, where the spirit dwells, all I really wanted was to find some intimacy, not just the fly-by-night sexual innuendoes Sam and I and then Tommy and I had. I wanted someone I could spend my life with and grow old with. I wanted someone to love me for my flaws, which I knew to be many.

Was there someone like that? My mother had always told me that God has someone special for each of us, that we must be patient, vigilant, and when the time is right, we will meet. But how does one arrange for one of these meetings? I wanted to know—yesterday! When Anne dropped me off after practice that night, I felt a sense of hope. I could not have been happier had I found a gold mine.

My other good friend, Joanne, who had recently retired after many years as a legal secretary, who had spent years without a partner or husband, married an eighty-five-year-old widower named Paul who lived in town just around the corner from where I lived. She invited me to come get grapefruit off their trees whenever I wanted. She spent the next five most delightful years of her life decorating his house and having dinner parties. He was waiting for her, and by the size of the rock she had on her ring finger, he really wanted her too. Before rehearsal was over on the evening after she got it, every woman in the choir had admired it. Joanne was lit up like Christmas on the town square.

As for Anne, I hate to even think how unfair life had been for her. She was such a help to me, and here, after less than a year of marriage, she became painfully aware that her husband came from a family with gay parents. But most apparent, they were not at all spiritually connected. She did eventually meet and marry the right guy. They even adopted a little girl named Mary. Her new husband's name is Barry, and they live in the state of Washington.

Yes, it was the coldest winter I had experienced in Naples. Joanne got married in February, and to add more misery to my circumstances, my beloved farmer of a grandfather, George Allen, died of heart failure in the Carlisle, Pennsylvania hospital. Anne was lassoed to her dunce of a guy in April. Next it was my turn; I could feel it. But first I had to get ready to fly back to Pennsylvania. I was not real keen on being back to live under the same roof with Mother, but I needed a little mothering, nurturing, and healing. I was sick to my soul, and I wanted my family. Somehow I had to put aside my judgments of them and go home.

I decided to get home by the quickest means possible, which meant flying. I sold a good many things, including my precious, heavy metal Brothers sewing machine. I was afraid it was too heavy to put on a plane. Now how rational was that decision! I regretted it in the end. Most newer-model machines are structured of lightweight vinyl or plastic and make it difficult to sew heavier fabrics. I spent all of April and through May 26 saying my farewells. There were tears and broken hearts, two in particular.

My friend Margaret had worked in downtown Naples over those five years, and we had many a happy lunch on the beach together or a stroll down Fifth Avenue. Margaret had a way of scooping me out of my loneliness and dejection when I needed it. So many times she had me come out to her home for a meal and some good company. She would invite me, and I would call a short time beforehand to say I couldn't make it when really I was just in one of my many *moods* and supreme discomfort. When this happened, I simply did not want to spread bad humor, the kind that leaves even the best-prepared meal feeling like a lump in the gut. Another thing was that Margaret's husband, Tom, had a way of scaring the daylights out of me at times. He drank too much, and one Thanksgiving, in a drunken stupor, he grabbed his shotgun and was wheeling it around the house like he was going to shoot someone. In my eyes, given what she lived with, besides two wonderful children, she was a saint. I especially hated saying good-bye to her.

The last I had seen of ole' Tommy after witnessing some of the destruction he left behind at the marina was him driving a very old, rickety milk delivery truck. It suited him. I did not like myself for taking off to get away from him the way I did. I mean, after all, he had supported me generously throughout my year of nurse's training. But he scared me. I know it was just a dream that warned me, but dreams do tell. I was not going to wait around for the first blow to hit. That would have been just plain stupid. And to think, I even considered marrying him. Had I married him, it would have only served to placate my guilty conscience for living with him out of wedlock. Considering what was in store for me next, I am so glad I didn't tie the knot.

Leaving also meant saying good-bye to Papa Gus, who had been watching over me like an angel ever since my accident. He said he could not let me go unless I allowed him to take me out once more for a meal. In fact, he came to church one Sunday to hear me sing. Afterward he escorted me to his old Pontiac, and we drove to the Holiday Inn Restaurant. He even came around and opened my car door for me. There were a lot of after-church diners that day. As we sat waiting for our roast beef and mashed potatoes, Gus looked at me with such endearing intent. I saw tears come to his eyes as he asked, "Sylvia, I guess there is nothing I can say to get you to stay, is there?" We toasted each other with glasses full of chilled ice tea. His eyes told me the tender heart in him was ripping in two. We both knew we would never see each other again. After all, he was eighty-six years old and often gasping for air from emphysema.

"Gus," I replied, "you have been so good to me. But right now I just need my family."

I heard his voice waver as he asked, "Will you marry me?"

"Gus," I said "I will come back to visit you, whenever and as much as I can."

He knew and I knew he very well might not be there anymore. He had breathed about his last from those old lungs.

"Gus," I said, gulping down some of my own tears, "if you believe in an afterlife as I do, you have to promise me you will not forget me to the Creator when you get there. I'm going to need a ticket to get in, do you think?" We laughed together.

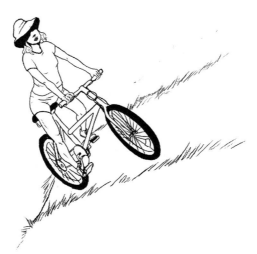

CHAPTER 4

Mile-High Hill

I left Naples feeling I had been let down. The hope I had when I first came was dashed to the ground. Now I knew it was just another town, only this one was full of multimillionaires, retirees, and people just passing through. Those passing through were a lot like me—hopefuls, finding out there was no pot of gold waiting for them. The most endearing part of Naples was the sweetness of that Gulf breeze. Even many of those who had found their pot of gold were drinking themselves to death. Or they were disillusioned with life and sick, often just waiting to die. The latter were the ones I often cared for in the hospital, trying to inject some enthusiasm—some desire to live—into them. But once a person gives up inside, there is not a lot that can be done for him or her physically. There were young people, but they were the ones just passing through. Eligible guys were few and far between. I was too sick with pain on most days to really care anyway.

Alcoholics had occupied just about every other room on the third floor of the hospital. Many of them were shackled to the bed to keep them from bolting. One man, I recall, had not been shackled. Even though he was the retired CEO and founder of a gin-manufacturing company, to look at him, he was just a scruffy, unshaven old man. I had just checked in on him one afternoon and was in the next room helping another patient when I looked out the window. My chin dropped at what my eyes beheld: he was flying down the street as fast as his long, skinny legs could carry him, hospital gown open and flapping in the breeze, bare butt exposed for the world to behold. The police picked him up at the corner pharmacy, where he was glugging down bottles of aftershave. Now, what would drive a person to this much desperation? Surely there was more to his life than alcohol. Whatever it was, it had him a prisoner in an iron fist.

I am no one to speak of drunken desperation, to judge the person resorting to alcohol for some peace of mind, or for maybe just even a little company at the bottom of a can of beer. For weeks before my departure from Naples, I had been bringing six-packs to my little breezeway room on weekends and once again, drinking myself into a stupor. But now I felt so alone, so totally alone. The day of departure could not come soon enough.

I sold what few pieces of furniture I had acquired for my little room—mostly a desk and office chair. The blue Raleigh had seen better days, especially since the accident, so I bought a new, lightweight, ten-speed Raleigh touring bike, a red one no less. Bill Hemmer helped me box it up for the flight. There would be no return trip by bicycle. I was, however, planning a trip to Lander, Wyoming, shortly after getting back to Pennsylvania. The Hemmers' son, Billy, had attended the National Outdoor Leadership School there. I at least had that to look forward to. Marjorie and Bill both took me to the airport on the morning of May 27, 1977. For whatever lay ahead, and for whatever new adventure I was to experience, it was time. I felt sadness at leaving such good friends behind, but also I felt a little spark of hope. As I prayed, "Oh God, let this be Thy will, not mine," a sense of peace washed over me.

> *Wheel going around and around, clicking, spinning, driving me further into life, away from, toward. Where have I begun, where have I been, where am I going? I just keep pedaling, around and around … I saw what I saw, I see what I see, I will see what there is to see. Oh, wheel going around and around, clicking, spinning, driving me further,*

further, further … When I stop, nobody knows; where I
stop I know not either. I just am, I just am, I … just … am.
I … am … I am … I … I … I … am … am … am …

The closer I got to home, the more I began to feel a deep hole open up inside me—a hole I had felt many times. Something was missing in me. I had a bizarre picture of myself in my mind of landing in Bogotá, Columbia, of all places. In the vision I was an accomplished nurse with her little cap perched on hair neatly pinned back into a bun. I was wearing a blue woolen nurse's cape that was blowing in the wind as I stepped out of the big plane and began my descent into a life married to, of all people, Alfonso. Now where do you think this image came from? It was really just part of my tormented thinking.

A few months before leaving, I had gotten a letter from him with a queen of hearts playing card in it. I could not believe my mother had given him my Florida address. I know she meant well. She wanted me married and with children, even if it meant marrying this foreigner for whom I had no feelings. Alfonso had pursued me for eight years of my miserable life. To me, he was like the devil waiting at the back door. And I had such a deep ache in my being. Life was one long, ongoing nightmare, a bad dream from which I could not awaken.

While I was away, my sister took what had been my bedroom, and with Grandma spending months at a time in our home when she was not at my Aunt Aileen and Uncle Chet's in Georgia, the spare room with a powder room became hers. I did not feel at all put out. I had put myself out five years ago. Besides, if there were to be any privacy for me in our family home, the basement bedroom was the place. However, there was not to be much privacy, because on the very first Saturday morning at 7:00 a.m., I heard Mother's sing-song voice from the top of the stairs, *"Sylvia, it's time to get up …"*

Oh, drat!

The expedition with the outdoor leadership school was to be a month long. I loved nature, and this school taught not only leadership and survival skills but ecology and wilderness preservation too. I had equipment to gather as well as the appropriate clothing, like shoes with Vibram soles, wool socks, and garments that could be peeled off or added on for easy

118

adjustments to climate change. If I got nothing else from the experience, I prayed it would give me a much-needed new perspective on life, perhaps some new direction. Before anything else, however, I needed to feel two wheels spinning beneath me.

My new bicycle with its ten speeds would take some learning to get it right as far as where the two levers were to be for the speed I wanted relative to ascending or descending. I rode the crest of the hill that made up my parents' development and then shifted into high to take the nearly mile-long descent from the top of Paxtang Avenue to the little town below. The warm May breeze whisked my hair back against my head, clearing my thoughts. At the bottom I carefully crossed the road and prepared to sprint back to the top. I miscalculated, briefly experiencing a familiar feeling of confusion. I failed to take into account that I had spent the last five years cycling at sea level, where the air was dense with oxygen and there were no hills. It took four stops to catch my breath and slow the rapid beat of my heart to get to the top. Oh dear, I felt like I was ninety. And was I ever to feel the kind of magic I felt with Sam, especially those few hours we spent together in Naples? The going was all … up … hill … now.

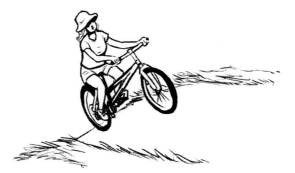

I took the train out West to Laramie, Wyoming, where I was loaded onto a rickety old school bus to get up to Lander. I knew nothing of what lay ahead. Soon I found myself, like the other twenty-two group members, loaded with what felt like a fifty-pound backpack. This, we were told, was "traveling light." We were taught everything from how to dig a hole for a toilet and then cover it to look like it had not been disturbed to where to camp at night to avoid being victims of avalanches or "widow makers," which were rotted trees ready to fall on us while we were sleeping. We learned how to read a topographical map by observing the placement of ridges in relation to waterfalls, streams, and rocks. We ate greens for lettuce, collected from streams, and even baked bread in special frying pans that could be turned one over the other and topped with coals to evenly distribute heat, forming a kind of campfire oven. We took turns, first the women and then the men, taking icy baths in Bomber Lake, a glacier lake named thus after a World War II bomber pilot flew into that mountain range in Roosevelt National Park and never flew out again. Brrr … But as fate would have it, something happened to me only four days into the thirty-day expedition.

We were, one-by-one, forming a line to cross over a roaring stream by stepping on large rocks. Jenny was in front of me, Kevin behind. I was about mid-stream when my foot slipped on the next rock. In order to not let my heavy backpack send me hurtling down into the rapids below, I stooped down for more control. I felt what could only be described as lightning searing through my left knee. I soon realized there was no way I could stand back up, especially with the load on my back. So, Todd, one of the team leaders, crossed back to where I was marooned, and Rick came in from the other side. Together they were able to help me stand up. Wounded, but so glad to finally be on solid ground, I breathed a prayer of thanksgiving and praised my helpers. But something was obvious immediately: my left knee, weakened from my bike accident in Florida, was not good.

Not much could be done for me out there in the wilderness of Wyoming. All they could do was take a good bit of the weight out of my pack. I used a bent but sturdy walking stick. Still, my knee was swollen and painful. Eighteen-year-old Andy was behind me while sixteen-year-old Sean was in front of me as we slowly ascended into the mountains. The higher we got, the more my sea-level lungs wheezed. I heard Sean say, "Can't you stop all that noise?" Both young men were my tent mates at night. Andy was a pretty decent young man, and so was Sean, even though he irritated me to the core. One day he contemplated trading one of our baking potatoes for a chew of tobacco from one of the leaders. At least he had the decency to ask me what I thought about the proposed transaction. I answered, "Hell, no!"

The next day we came to an area of numerous jutting cliffs, where everybody but me used carabineers and ropes to practice climbing. I was grateful not to have to do this exercise. I sat quietly nearby, observing, thinking to myself, *Sylvia, what are you doing out here? You can take the girl out of the city, but you can't take the city out of the girl.* And the further we ascended that first week, the more trouble I had breathing. And by twelve and thirteen thousand feet, I was throwing up and shitting between the rocks.

Seven days into the expedition, we mounted a place called Goat Flat. Here we learned the dynamics of what to do in case of a lightning storm in a high place. We were to get as flat to the ground and as far away from the metal of our backpacks as possible. Three days after this, one leader and one group member were able to hike me out over a ridge and back down to a pickup point. There, the van took me all the way back to Lander. The beauty of the mountains and reservations took my breath away, but I had had enough. I cried tears of relief, along with some sadness at having to leave the people I had grown close to, even if it had been only ten days instead of the full month-long experience.

Back in Lander, I saw a doctor at the clinic in town. They took x-rays of my knee and gave me crutches. I soaked in a hot tub before going to bed, and the next morning I caught the bus to Laramie. The train slowly took me east—back to where life was familiar. Still, that hole in my soul left me with a feeling of foreboding defeat: *"You'll never make it, Sylvia."* My stomach churned at the thought of being back in my mother's house. I was sad and angry, and it was dark all around me. Who turned out the lights? Most folks, when they saw me or spoke to me, did not see the darkness, but it was behind me, in me, and before me. Days and nights ran together. I put one foot in front of the other; what else could I do?

THE *PLAN*

As the daughter of successful business people, I was instilled with the desire to be self-sufficient. Mother and Father wanted me to find a spouse, to have children and a life, but if ever the need should arise, I needed to be self-sufficient too. This was the basis of my impetus, my plan. Unfortunately, no one knew the difficulty I was having keeping my ducks in a row. Easy tasks had a way of becoming not so easy when I set about trying with every ounce of my being to complete them. For a simple example, as a teenager I had to mow the lawn in front of our house.

I set about mowing from the sidewalk to the house, to the sidewalk to the house … sidewalk … house … sidewalk … Until the neighbor yelled out to me over the hum of the mower, "Why don't you mow the length of the yard?" I think I felt a little embarrassed, not having figured it out for myself. This may sound simplistic, but multiply it by twenty-nine years of dysfunctional challenges, and it makes for a great deal more work than necessary. I knew something was wrong with my logic, but I could not figure out what. As part of wanting to be self-sufficient, I planned on going to the University of Pennsylvania in Philadelphia. I mean, I knew I wasn't dumb. However, in preparation for this I also felt the need to buck up, so to speak, on my sense of logic. I had already taken and passed college algebra, but what could it hurt to repeat it?

My hope was that taking algebra would improve my cognitive skills, so I signed up for that and, of all things, swimming for the second semester of the summer. That way I would also meet people. "Gregarious" should have been my middle name. I had a very strong innate desire to be with people.

On top of school, I figured I'd best prove my independence by getting a job—you guessed it—at the hospital. Any reasonable person would have gotten the message that the heavy labor was adding to my difficulties, but I was clueless. I worked on the orthopedic department, lifting heavy casts and equipment. It was even more taxing than the Florida work. It wiped me out. The bathroom stalls were the only place where I could pour out my true feelings, the feelings that said to me, *Sylvia, you are certainly dying at this.* I didn't listen to my own inner voice. I just kept on keeping on, perpetrating the damage I had already done myself and sending myself deeper into a hole I was digging—my own grave, it seemed.

Being a people lover posed a different kind of problem for someone my age. People would tell me their names, and invariably within five minutes I could not repeat it. This problem with my short-term memory had been with me from the time I was very young. The little "I can't remember" demon was with me as a candy striper at the old folks' home, and it was just one more source of embarrassment.

When I was ten, someone told me the name of a tree, the leaf of which I had in my hand. It was a gingko leaf. A few minutes later, Mother asked, "Now, can you tell me the name of that tree again?" When I gave her a puzzled look, she continued, "Are you that dumb?" I obviously was impacted by these words from Mother since I remember it all these years later. But I was right about one thing: I was going to meet people, even that someone special, by going back to school.

One fine day toward the end of July, I had just come from swim class, my short blonde hair wet and mussed. I was wearing a bright orange Wheaties sweatshirt. I sat down at a big, round table in the student union cafeteria. Ten of us sat around jabbering about this, that, or the other thing. Two of the girls were wooing a cute guy in the chow line. I remember thinking how childish they seemed—don't they know that is no way to get a guy? But I was twenty-nine and unmarried. Who was I to give out mating tips? Only two of us were not part of the crowd because suddenly they all got up and walked out, leaving just me and a quiet young man sitting across the table from me. I got up and moved closer, and he did the same. He had such a pleasant, inquiring expression on his face. His name was Don, better known as Donnie in his hometown of Shamokin, Pennsylvania.

Don had been in the army until 1970. He served two years in Vietnam, building bridges and cutting roads through the jungle. As I looked into his eyes, it was difficult imagining him wielding an M16 rifle—but that's what they did. They only lost one comrade, a new recruit who lost it out of fear, committing suicide. I saw tears come to Don's eyes. When he got off the bus in Sunbury, returning home, no one threw a parade for him, nor did we celebrate for any of these lads who had been through so much. Still, Don was proud of his service. The conversation went on for maybe ten minutes. But the next day and every school day for the rest of the summer, we looked for each other in the cafeteria.

Don was severely hard of hearing, like his father and brother. Each time we met, he would watch my face intently, trying to pick up my words. He was just getting used to a hearing aid and was frustrated with what seemed like a whole different world of sound to him. It was the world of the deaf and hard of hearing. But there we sat, day after day, looking into each other's faces, soaking up the intimacy. This was what I was waiting for. This young man, with his somewhat rounded, endearing face, was here for me. Things did not really take off for us, however, until October.

We were at a familiar place, near the vending machines in the cafeteria where we met, when he asked, "Would you care to go to the school hay ride tomorrow night?" I felt my heart swoon, like he had asked me to a prom. He was to be in Pittsburgh that day for his work, but he was going to call me when he got back. I waited by the phone all afternoon, watching it, ready to pick up on a heartbeat. Several of my mother's calls came in, and it was getting dark. Finally, at five o'clock the phone rang; it was him.

He picked me up in his beautiful canary-yellow Camaro. It was a bitter cold night for a hayride, but snuggled together in the hay, we were like baby birds in a sunny, warm nest. I listened to Don's pleasant voice sing "Ninety Nine Bottles of Beer" throughout most of the slow ride around the farm. It was not my favorite song, but he seemed to be enjoying it. I figured him for a light drinker, because he didn't have a beer belly. In fact, he had a nice body, one that felt good close to me. After the ride through moonlit fields, the party of maybe twenty-five fellow students gathered around a huge bonfire for marshmallows and hot chocolate. He stood closely behind me, wrapping a blanket around me, shielding me from the cold. I felt complete, like this person behind me was making up for a part of me that had not been there before.

Don came for supper the next night. Mother and Father just had to meet this special young man. Don shared he had just completed Diet Workshop and had gotten his weight down some significant pounds. God bless my mother—she smiled and said, "Well good for you. Here, have some more mashed potatoes." Then she made sure he had another pork chop or two.

Months later, after I started cooking for him, she was telling me, "You need to start feeding him less."

"Well, Mom," I should have said. "You are the one who started putting the pounds back on him." She even made a point of coming over and making sure we had a dish of fresh vegetables in the refrigerator.

By December, the two of us had gotten pretty close. One night we were out bar hopping until we found a Mexican one with live music. We came back to the house at one or two in the morning. I don't know if it was all the alcohol in our blood or the closeness again—probably both—but we sat there on the couch in the living room baring our souls to each other. I told him about my experience with the young man who took me on the ride of my life, stealing cars and television sets all across the country. I could see the shock effect of my ranting on Don's face. Then, to my surprise, he also shared something about himself that I knew was very personal. Somehow it felt safe, like I knew he would not judge me, or I him, for such folly.

Early the next day, Sunday, I awoke with a start, the alcohol drained from my system. And with the jolt of wakefulness, I did a sudden reality check. Why on earth did I tell him so much about what happened with Sam and me? Surely I ruined my chances with this marvelous man. I might as well have told him I was really a man dressed as a woman. Why, why, why? I quickly dressed and ventured out into the frosty air, walking and walking until I found myself at the mall two miles from home. I wandered aimlessly, staring into nothingness until finally going to a phone, plopping in a couple of quarters, and calling him.

"Don," I said, "are we still together?"

"Well, yeah," he replied. "What makes you think any differently?"

I told him how ashamed I was of having run away with that fellow. He laughed lightly and said, "We've all done things we regret—everyone has. We're okay."

I breathed a long, full sigh of relief. Twenty minutes later, his familiar yellow Camaro pulled up outside. I was never so glad to see anyone in my life—especially this someone. This guy was special, and I knew it down deep in my soul.

A week before Christmas, we were at his apartment one evening, wrapped in each other's arms, fixed on a precious moment together. Don looked deeply into my eyes and said, "Sylvia, I want you to marry me, but I am stuck on what my brother is going through. I just cannot get into a place like where he is." He had a brother who was in a miserable, dysfunctional marriage to a woman who used him to exert her seemingly deep hatred over an ex-husband or possibly even a hatred for men in general.

By now I too felt the struggle his brother was having. He was barely able to afford an ounce of self-respect. Of course there are always two or more sides to a story, but the man could barely speak without her cutting him down and demeaning his gentle character. I could feel Don struggling with this, so I said, "Don, if you like we can set a date, let's say, for a year from our first date in October. If it gets too uncomfortable, we will postpone it or just cancel all together."

This must have been all it took, because now we were officially engaged— with no diamond and only the mere mentioning of our engagement to family. Surely the delight was registering on our faces.

The highlight of many of our weekends was trips back and forth from Harrisburg to Shamokin. Being with Don's mother was a little like stepping under a microscope. I knew she was evaluating this potential daughter-in-law. I remember saying how good her roast smelled cooking in the kitchen, and she looked at me as if to say, "Can I really believe you? Or are you just making conversation?" Nope, no one was going to pull a fast one on her—especially with her baby, Donnie. Everyone seemed to love Don for who he was, their *Donnie*, more than where he had been or what he had done. He was the youngest of three siblings. His sister, his brother in the next town up, and everybody was small town proud. Clearly Shamokin had seen better days.

Living in a depressed coal town was not easy for anyone, especially Don's sister, who lived in the next township with her three children and the absence of a caring husband. I saw immediately how wounded she was. She had to be totally there for those children in addition to staying by the coal furnace. If she was out of the house too long, the coals grew cold. She knew firsthand what it meant to have to "pick coal from off the railroad tracks" to provide warmth to their little house, which had no bathroom and only a toilet in the basement. She, like Don—excuse me, *Donnie*—who had experienced this with his sister-in-law, knew what it was like to have someone call her at three in the morning to complain about family. The woman who called was her husband's lover, but this irate woman did not have to tell Don's sister what a two-timer her husband was. She knew that, and her pain was deep; I felt it.

Even though I was under Mom Deppen's constant evaluation, I started to feel like one of the family. I knew what depression felt like; nobody had to tell me. Saturday mornings we would walk downtown for the street-side market and the row of businesses that had roughed the down times. Shamokin had thrived as a coal town, but now it was failing miserably. Don and I would go into Jones Hardware to get a plumbing part to fix the toilet in Mom's bathroom, or we would meander through the Fun Shop, taking in the cards and showcases of gifts, including everything from dolls to a miniature coal-shoveling Derek. We would end the morning at Coney Island, where we got burgers loaded with mustard and onions, finally coming home smelling like conies ourselves. We brought Mom one, and I saw the half smile on her face as she bit into it, an onion caught in the corner of her mouth. Life in Shamokin *was* a coney.

On our first Christmas together, Mom had Don and I go to her attic, where Don showed me his dad's pea coat from when he had served in the navy. He showed it to me with a sense of pride that only a person who had himself served his country could know. We brought down the long, cardboard box containing a four-foot artificial tree and set it up in the living room. I could tell it had been around for quite a few years because the stand at the bottom was worn and loose. Don helped put each ornament on it with the care of a son who had done it many times for his mother. We were family already, and the wedding was supposedly eleven months away.

Those months went quickly, and by April plans were shifting quickly too. The wedding was planned for July 15. Who could wait another six months? We were on a roll, and at the helm was—who else?—my mother. My brother had married in 1976, and now Mother was caught up in what every mother dreams of—her daughter being married. My sister, bless her heart, seemed to always be left behind. She had just had her heart broken by a young man named Randy, and now she was in a relationship with a younger fellow who was even less attentive. The young man, Brian, worked with her at Longenecker's Hatchery in Elizabethtown, and they would sit on the back stoop at midday eating lunch together. One day she asked for a sip of his lemonade, and he replied heartlessly, "No." But now Wendy seemed delighted with the plans for my wedding, knowing her turn would come.

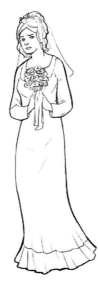

Mother's idea of planning was, "This is how we are going to do this, no exceptions." I was expected to reply, "Yes, Mother." One Saturday afternoon, Grandma, Mother, Aunt Aileen, and I, with Father in the background, were having a strategic discussion about the wedding. The debate was whether we wanted the reception at this restaurant or that hotel. I insisted on having bouquets for each of the bridesmaids, while Mother thought that too extravagant.

One thing was certain: Rev. MacPherson, from my grandparents' church, was to do the ceremony. I had loved this man, who had a gentle Irish brogue, since I was a little girl visiting the farm and we went to the Presbyterian Church in Mechanicsburg. I still felt like that little girl standing behind the pew in the fourth row from the front, my eyes closed and clutching the program while listening to his musical voice and with the organist playing quietly in the background. Then the talk switched to where we were going to have the wedding, in a church or in a natural setting. I loved being out in nature, so I decided to try and have it at a place called Ranchland.

The planning was about over for the afternoon when Don finally came onto the scene. We were sitting together on the porch swing outside Mother's kitchen when I told him everything we had been discussing. When it came to the place for the wedding and I told him about Ranchland, I felt a distinct chill come into the air. You would have thought icicles were hanging from the gutter.

"Sylvia," I heard him say, "I wish I could have been in on this little talk you ladies were having. Don't I get a say?"

I was getting my first taste of Don's "let's do it together" theme for our marriage, the very insistence that eventually became the cement that would hold our lives together firmly. I did a quick reality check. Then I wanted to say, "You mean it is not all up to Mother? Wow, what a new concept." I just smiled to myself, realizing I would soon be out from under *her* roof. I would have this man, 24/7, helping to break Mother's controlling clutches. Yes! However, I would soon find out she wasn't done yet.

I was to wear a simple, floor-length, country-style dress I found in a in a McCall's pattern catalogue, and I was determined to make it myself. However, by this time I was having so much back pain from my accident years prior that I struggled to sit at the sewing machine. My backache left me, too often, curled in a ball on my bed in the basement. By March

I ended up having to even quit my job at the hospital. It was all too much on my already overtaxed brain. Then there was the matter of my mother upstairs, running the show. She was quickly becoming the wicked witch of the east in *The Wizard of Oz*. However, June rolled around and I was still a lump in that big old bed, the very bed her old cat, Rusty, had chosen to do his business on in rebellion of my homecoming. The dress lay in pieces all over that desolate room. Again, dear ol' Mom came to the rescue. She had the wife of a business associate finish it for me. *Oh, poo.* This was one more exertion of my weak willfulness.

In the meantime, Don was readying himself for the big day. His brother, David, was to be his best man, and his friend Mike, from Shamokin, was to stand for him, along with Billy from down the road in Trevorton. The photographer we hired was a man everyone called Old Mose, for Moses. He had taken our engagement photo, and he interested Don in doing some photography for him at the same time. Don had gotten his first good camera while in Vietnam and wanted to go professional. I spent a lot of time posing for him in front of different homemade backdrops in our tiny apartment in Camp Hill.

The day of the wedding could not come quickly enough. As we drove into Ranchland, I felt really silly for having insisted on all the flowers from a florist because the fields all around the place were filled with beautiful day lilies. I could have picked my fill of flowers and then some. My sister and cousin, Carolyn, and friend, Linda, and I were all dressed in our little country outfits, which were probably more suited to a barn dance. Father came in for some photos in front of the big stone fireplace in the lodge. I remember thinking, *Shouldn't I be feeling something?* I honestly felt like one of the foolish brides in Christ's parable of the seven wise and seven foolish bridesmaids. I could not help feeling all the oil in my lamp was used up. I was taking too much Vicodin to feel much of anything except scared.

As Father took me down the aisle, the flower girl, Don's niece Crystal, was swinging from a nearby willow tree. The congregation of family and friends were a blur. When I finally stood next to Don and it was time to say my part of the vows, I opened my mouth and absolutely nothing came out but a gasp. Wendy nudged me a bit before I could get it out, "I do." The whole wedding felt surreal.

By the time I got into my prince's chariot, the Camaro, I breathed a sigh of relief. We were alone at last. We spent one night in the Pentagon

Inn outside Washington DC, and the next day took off for Miami and a four-day honeymoon in the Bahamas. As we got off the plane in Nassau, my bad knee locked. Don practically carried me into the terminal. How could such an occasion feel any less romantic? I must have been popping Vicodin the whole time. I was even oblivious to the sex. To be honest, I did not like it, but if it meant being close to Don then it was all right.

That first evening, Don struggled persistently to get the film in my brother's underwater camera un-jammed so he could take some pictures snorkeling. I saw what a patient, persistent man I had married. Later, he set up a video camera on the porch of our villa and shot a few frames of us slopping mango into each others' mouths, juice dripping off our elbows and onto the floor. We had a dinner of lobster. There was a satisfied grin on Don's face, and the butter dripped off his chin. We spent the next day lounging around the resort hotel and beach and riding bicycles all over Nassau. The whole time my sore knee was aching like I was a seventy-year-old instead of a newlywed. Little did I know how I would test Don's blessed patience, how my desire not to feel pain would color the whole first twenty-four years of our marriage.

We got back to the Camp Hill apartment on a Friday, so I had him with me the weekend yet before he had to returned to work. On that first Saturday together, I made a pot of coffee strong enough to make our hair stand up. We took a long, long walk that first morning, taking in the many big homes in the area. Ours was just a tiny second-floor house apartment. Of course I had to have the little tabby cat there too that I had acquired since getting home from Florida. That little guy, taken from his mother too soon, almost got us thrown out one night.

The landlord and his wife lived on the first floor of the house, and a young girl by the name of Kim lived in the front apartment across from us upstairs. One night Peewee got locked outside. He stood under our bedroom window screaming for someone to let him in. The next day, we got the cold shoulder from the landlord as he complained of being awakened by our cat. I must have been having a run on deep sleep, and of course Don, without his hearing aids, heard nothing. Neither of us heard his desperate cries. After that, if he was not in the house at bedtime, I started leaving the lower door ajar. One night, not too long after this, he brought a baby rabbit in and proceeded to eat it on the upper landing. Again, I heard nothing, but the next day Kim complained, "Your cat scared me to death. I thought a baby was being murdered on the landing!" Fortunately, not too long after this, we moved to our own home and could put in a cat door.

Don soon learned what a cat lady I was because we had them by the twos and threes. Now there are five, plus two basset hounds. Cats have always been such a comfort to me. They are sleek and graceful, and when I have been struggling inside over the years, they have come to my rescue over and over.

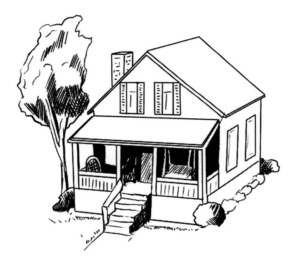

LITTLE HOUSE ON TWENTY-FOURTH STREET

Home buying was made easy by my blessed parents. But I was not about to make Don's life easy—not by a long shot. We rented a U-haul for the occasion and had friends help us pack box after box. I managed to forget leaving pizza bites in the oven at our old place, and the landlord didn't find them until there were three species of mold growing on them. We were certainly out of their graces. Those boxes sat for months in our dining room because I was too depressed to unpack them. The house felt like forty-degrees that first winter, and most of it was painted blue or purple inside, except for the living room that our friend George Bingaman helped paper with lovely green and white foliage. His wife, Betsy, brought her homemade goodies. We eventually painted the other rooms in our house to make the place more cheerful. However, I believe now there was a lot more to the chill I was feeling at the time. There was no doubt a ghost in this house, one that would make my misery even worse.

Before this I had struggled just with these *feelings*, but I had never been self-destructive. Now things were changing inside me. For one thing, I never quite recovered from having our daughter; it was getting darker and darker inside me. Our neighbors, Paul and Hazel, told us that the woman who had lived in the house originally had committed suicide there. Our daughter as a small child even saw what she could only describe later as a spirit or shadow in the night. But at the time we just dismissed it as a bad dream. It may not have been because I was getting seriously suicidal. Inside I simply did not want to live anymore. Fear and pain were crowding my conscious mind, till I could not think anymore. I could barely move some days, and I would lie around brooding. Finally my parents, who lived near us, had seen enough. Mother, to the rescue once again, found a doctor who used hypnosis to help people in their illnesses.

Dr. Jones' office was like any other practitioner's, except instead of being led into an exam room, I was led into his office. The rather tall, elderly doctor began to lead me into a trance, probably hoping to get to the bottom of where all my pain was coming from, but I was barely into it five minutes when I began to cry and cry and cry … I could not hold the sobs inside any longer. Realizing my desperation, he decided to stop the session. I must have sat there an hour trying to get my wits about me enough to drive home. He told me I needed to see someone else, more of a counselor. I was ready for something—anything but the way I was. The doctor gave me the name of a psychologist who worked for the prisons but saw people in his office at home for counseling.

Dr. Barton greeted me at the door that evening and led me to his office in the back. In his office I sat in a big leather chair while he sat at his desk. His walls were lined with credentials and books, and a globe with an eagle perched on top sat off to the side. We just talked for awhile. I didn't feel I had a whole lot to tell him, except that I was in this elusive state of pain. I had no idea what was causing it. Then he had me close my eyes and do some breathing and visualization. It was not some deep hypnotic state; I didn't want to go there again. It was just picturing myself in relaxing scenes, like in the woods or standing on a beach.

132

The sessions went on once a week for about two months, until out of exasperation I blurted out, "You know, none of this is really working. I am just in too much pain. I think I need to see someone else." I didn't want to be rude—I was just too deeply disturbed to even try his suggestions. So, as life would have it, I started going to a psychiatrist, a doctor who could "really fix this for me!"

When I started to see Dr. A in 1980, I had no idea it could go on as long as it did. But from that very first session I began to think he was *God*. Who else could listen to all the garbage I was unloading on him without saying a word? He just sat in his chair across from me while I sat in another big, soft leather chair emptying box after box of Kleenex, spilling my guts. When he pulled out his prescription pad that first time, I did not know how many times he would be writing those prescriptions. They must fell whole forests for psychiatrists, because it seemed like every time I went in he would up the dose or prescribe something different. I was about to become a walking pharmacy.

In the meantime, I was struggling along on a really bad knee. One surgeon took my whole knee apart and put it back together again. But when the arthritis set in a year later, it was ten times worse. I was literally going to hell in a hand basket because I felt like a ninety-year-old. Having ongoing, undiagnosed pain is a challenge for anyone, but when you put a little one in the mix, it feels impossible. I had to stay cheerful and engaged in our daughter's development, but all I wanted to do was mope around the house. Smiling was difficult for me because I had these strange spasms in my face. And carrying our daughter often gave me horrible chest pain. I honestly felt like I was dying inside.

On top of it all I was having woman problems because everything had dropped from my broken pelvis in 1974. I was lucky to even have had our daughter, Susan. But she became such a light in my life and Don's. I just had to make it. By 1981, I had a hysterectomy and some repair work to my bladder. A week after the surgery, I dragged myself back to Dr. A's office and what had become a kind of *confession booth*. I'm not Catholic, but that is what it felt like. I had never bared my soul quite like I did with this doctor. Well, on this particular evening I must have hit rock bottom, pain wise, because the words came out loud and clear, "I'm going to kill myself." I could not believe the words had come from my mouth!

That same evening I found myself being admitted for the first time to the psychiatric ward. It felt like the softest, safest place to fall. Inside I did not really know what I was going to do. I was just so desperate. Going home would mean the rigors of being a housewife, mother, and lover, and I just was not up to it. To make matters worse, I had even kept on drinking on top of the psych meds. Once I started drinking, it was hard to stop because the detox made the pain a hell of a lot worse. I would find myself between a rock and a hard place, struggling to stay conscious on top of the haze. Wet laundry stayed in the washer for days at a time. Cleaning was only an idea, not something I could easily start, much less finish. Sewing projects sat for months to be completed. And through it all, I was trying to hold part time nursing positions with agencies. I was a total wipeout, and I knew it. Now, here in the hospital, I did not have to think about any of that. I could be just little ol' me with my little ol' problems.

After only a few days in the hospital, with people regularly checking in on me, talk sessions every few hours, meds administered, and meals being served on a tray, I was ready to go home. I don't think the words, "I feel better" came out of my mouth, but my conscience ate at me. I had to buck up and be the woman I was meant to be. When I left the hospital the first time, I simply felt stronger, not really better at all. In time I had two back surgeries on top of the hysterectomy, and most painful of all, seven knee surgeries. Nobody wanted to give someone so young an artificial knee. I was stuck wrapping it with a bandage and a brace and limping hither and yon. Nothing really worked. I would limp horribly trying to walk our Dalmatian dog, Ranger. He was the dog from hell because he could not stop rearranging my house. I simply did not need the chaos. I had enough on my mind just living.

The drinking progressed to whole weekend binges. We would take our little Sun Ray camper every year to Knoebel's Grove over Labor Day, enjoying the park and sitting around campfires with our daughter and her good friend, Teresa. But I often sent Don off with the girls while I stayed back quietly sipping Budweiser. The melancholy grew like clouds before a hurricane. I know now the alcohol only exacerbated my melancholy, but the more down I felt in the '80s and early '90s, the more I wanted to drink. And the more I drank, the more I was admitted to the hospital.

Now the hospital admissions were becoming regular as I spiraled downward. In 1982, I made my first very real attempt at suicide, the one that almost ended my life. I swallowed two bottles of antidepressants and was on life support in the hospital. When I got home, I picked right up with the drinking. I was beginning to not care about anything. I quite literally had the spine of a cod, but this fish didn't want to swim anymore. She was tired, broken, writhing from the beatings life still seemed to be inflicting. I was afraid to go on living. It didn't seem worth it. I was becoming a zombie.

By 1985 I had been admitted several times to the psych ward, once at a place called Phil Haven. This was an all-new experience for me. It was a big place, set at the edge of the woods in Mt. Gretna, Pennsylvania. I felt I was a long way from home, even though I had once lived thousands of miles away in Florida. I felt more lost than ever. The people were kind. They talked to me regularly, like at Polyclinic, the meals were good, and as usual I fit right in. But I didn't want to be there at all. *Take me home, God, please take me home.* I was so forlorn that I wanted to go outside and get lost in the woods. That way I felt I would at least be close to God. But the doors were locked and the ward secured. No one dared wander off.

After two weeks I was sent home with a prescription for the twelve steps of Alcoholics Anonymous in my hand. There were meetings all over my hometown of Harrisburg. My first meeting was a Sunday-evening speaker meeting in the cafeteria of the hospital across the river. It was set with numerous tables and chairs and people milling around, conversing like they were family and close friends. I felt welcome before anyone even spoke to me. I wondered what all the gab was about. I had been isolated a long time, and even though others were reaching out to me, I wondered if I really wanted to be there. The meeting began promptly at seven. Then I heard the words I needed to hear—not that I was ready, but I listened—"We came to believe that we were powerless over alcohol, and our lives had become unmanageable." The *unmanageable* part struck me the most. I knew deep down that this was exactly where I needed to be.

The next meeting was at noon above a soup kitchen in downtown Harrisburg. This meeting was smaller and in more of a living room setting. There were big, overstuffed chairs and couches, some of them worn and tattered. I could tell some of the people were from shelters and off the street while some were state workers from the nearby offices. And instead of a speaker meeting, it was a closed discussion group; in other words, you had to belong to the club. Again, *How It Works* was read, followed by some rules and regulations known as their *Traditions*. I was hearing what I needed to hear, but inside I must have still been the gullible, swayable little girl, because that evening I mentioned to Mother, "Mother, I'm an alcoholic."

She replied, "But you can't be an alcoholic. We don't have any alcoholics in the family." So, as fate would have it, I stopped going.

With the early '90s came a knee replacement. Let me tell you, if you don't like pain, I don't recommend this kind of surgery. But in the long run it was a saving grace for me. Finally I had two functioning legs. I could throw away the ace bandages, canes, and crutches. I was not all that graceful at first. I felt like I was walking on a wooden leg from so much surgery on it. But now I felt sure I was going to get my life back with no more pain. Ha, what a joke. I was fooling myself, and even after fully accepting my new knee, I continued to bellyache to Dr. A about the misery, the elusive, *never put your finger on it P-A-I-N.* The pill cocktails were still being poured. In 1991 he wrote a prescription for a medicine called Klonopin, a narcotic tranquilizer.

I was to take two milligrams of the Klonopin three times a day, but I loved the stuff and would pop an extra one into my mouth regularly. When I wasn't sloughing around the house, I was in panic mode. I was a disaster in the grocery store and a dangerous woman with a credit card, running up hundreds and hundreds of dollars on *things* I thought would make me happy. And through it all I writhed—I just could not stop moving—and picked my fingers until they were raw and bleeding. Nothing seemed to be helping. After a while, I became so intoxicated from the Klonopin that I would fall all the time. I fell down the basement steps twice. In 1993, I made one of my messiest attempts at suicide.

With a whole bottle of Klonopin in my pocket I went to the Top's Bar and Grill. But I was only interested in the bar. I sat drinking long enough to get up the courage for what I thought I had to do. I *had* to swallow those pills and get it over with. I had been to too many pain clinics and psych wards. I couldn't go on. The pain was too deep, and the sorrow and failure were too much to cope with. I just wanted to end it all. My husband and family would be much better off without me, or so I thought. I stumbled and fell on my way to the car, and once I was out there, I downed the pills.

I must have had reservations deep down inside, because a little later, in a blackout, I managed to drag myself back into the bar. I just laid there in the doorway unable to pick myself up. I heard the bartender say, "Lady, please don't die in my bar" just as I threw up the contents of my stomach onto the entryway. Soon I was in an ambulance and to my disappointment, still alive. I couldn't even commit suicide successfully. By now I had been on that psych ward so many times they practically had the door open with a sign on it, "Welcome back, Sylvia."

One morning in April of 1994, it was nine o'clock in the morning and I was already snorkeled from vodka and orange juice—several glasses—for breakfast. I was going to the state store for a new supply when I turned off Twenty-Eighth Street onto Walnut Street. Just as I turned, a lady stepped into the path of my car. I missed her by a thread. I had to pull to the side up ahead to gather my wits. That was the day I stopped drinking. It was bad enough what I was doing to my husband and daughter. Our family life was slowly and painfully degenerating to where our daughter stayed to herself upstairs and my husband prayed while he worked during the day that he would come home and find me alive. I was not going to kill someone with my drinking.

The only thing that held my life together were some God-given constants: a husband who believed in hard work and loved me dearly, in spite of it all; a daughter who got more beautiful with the years; my love of sewing—I could not hold my fingers still, so this skill helped a lot—and my desire to be with people to do the work I *thought* I was cut out to do. Yet every time I attempted nursing, agency after agency and nursing home after nursing home, I came out of the experience feeling frustrated and disappointed. The very idea of nursing was becoming repulsive to me. I would work so hard professionally and get nowhere. My resume was looking like a colorful wannabe collage until finally Dr. A helped get me on disability. Everybody thought this would be a good thing. I even thought so. But when I found myself sitting at home, depressed and anxious regardless of a steady Social Security check, things went from bad to worse.

Faith **Is the Bird**

Enlightenment: *"Faith is the bird that feels the
light, and sings in the dark before the dawn."*
—Tagore

I was on one of my regular vacations from life—yes, the psych ward at
Polyclinic—in 1995 when for some reason the clouds parted and I could
say officially that the depression had lifted. It happened as clearly and
distinctly as the day the curtain came down at my aunt and uncle's in New
Jersey thirty-seven years before. I have no real explanation for this, except
down deep now I felt a change was in store; I prayed there was. Something
was going to happen to put my life back on track. I could feel it. I was ready
for my star role in life, to do something, somewhere that would make a
difference, not just in my life but in the lives of others; something that was
meant to be. I wanted to be that idol of a person Mother and Father told
me I was meant to be.

I continued to trip into and out of the hospital. Even now, with my
slightly enlightened temperament, I continued to complain. Then in May
of 1998, again during one of my famous appearances at the hospital, an
elderly neurologist who had been following me for years, Dr. Brown, said
something that would change my life forever. He said, "Sylvia, you remind
me of someone who has fallen and hit her head." I had complained to him
so often of my head ringing and hurting, and by now I was also exhibiting
signs of nerve damage to my face. My tongue was dragging to the side so
much that it was causing me to choke easily and bite it while I was chewing.
What was happening to me now? I continued to withdraw in a kind of
mourning. I went home from the hospital this time with Dr. Brown's words
ringing in my head.

One morning shortly after getting home, I awoke very early with my
head ringing and hurting—it was getting old and tiresome—but on this
morning in particular, I thought to do something different. I went out to
the study in our dining room, and knowing Don would not hear me with
his hearing aids out for the night and Susan was all the way upstairs, I cried
out, "God, what happened to me? Why am I like this? I need to know."

The Dream

For now we see through a glass darkly,
but then we will see face to face.
—1 Corinthians 13:12

Two months later, I started to see a stairwell in the back of my mind. It was the stairwell right outside our kitchen door in the city apartment where I lived as a child. I didn't know why I was seeing this. Two weeks later, I again awoke early in the morning, but this time I relived falling head first into a nine-foot stairwell as a child. With a flash like a camera going off, it flooded my conscious mind. I saw it all, down to minute details. *Oh my God.* What *does it all mean?*

As It Happened

When I was six years old and in the first grade with Miss Tanler at Melrose, I had come home from school for lunch one day to find my brother and his friend, Jackie Nagle, playing on a ledge over an inner stairwell—not the one I had seen in the back of my mind outside the kitchen earlier. They were slowly working their feet way out onto the ledge with their hands on the opposite wall to steady themselves. Florida, our cleaning lady and a rather heavyset, robust woman who seconded as one of those sitters to us, was cleaning the windows in the French double doors by the tiled, concrete landing that laid ominously below. She turned long enough to chase the boys off the ledge. It was indeed treacherous. But she did not see me standing by the corner dish cabinet looking on intently, and thinking, *Oh ... that looked like fun.* When she turned back to her work, I slipped out onto that ledge, all the way out to the nine-foot drop. Then, to my horror, I was too small and my hands slipped down the wall. I fell head first into a bucket of scrub water she had sitting there, probably saving me from a broken neck. Instead I banged the back of my

head, creating years of havoc with a head injury and severely traumatizing my upper spine.

Florida turned to look once again, and she must have thought I fell off the bottom step into the bucket, because seeing me pull my dripping head out of the bucket sent her into one of her hardy belly laughs. But there was *nothing* funny about it! I was so horrified I ran up two flights of stairs, changed my dress, and dried my hair so Mother would not see what a *bad* thing I did. I came downstairs and sat at the table, and Mother put a bowl of steaming hot tomato soup and a grilled cheese sandwich on the table in front of me. It was my favorite, but it *all went on my lap*, scorching my thighs. I could not get it into my mouth. Mother came over to help me get cleaned off. She shook me a little and said, "*Sylvia, what is wrong with you?*" But I could not get the words out to tell her.

I again went upstairs and changed my dress and went off to school for the afternoon. The next thing I remembered was Miss Tanler kind of peeling my head off the desk. Again I heard the words, "*Sylvia, what is wrong with you?*" Again I could not put the words together to tell her. Mother came for me and I went home, where I proceeded to sleep for a week. Back then we did not go to the doctor if we were just a little *sick*, so I was on my own to just kind of sleep it off.

Who knows? I probably had a concussion. But now, in 1998, this new information posed a new problem. What, if anything, could be done to reverse the damage? Probably nothing, but I at least needed to do something to lighten the misery. What could I do? I, of course, shared all this with Dr. A, but even he seemed baffled by this sudden revelation. Was it a dream, or was it the real deal? Maybe he didn't know, but the important thing was ... I knew.

Given this information, Dr. A finally realized I must have been in some really severe pain. "*Hellooo ... what have I been trying to tell you the last eighteen years?*" So he started me on—what else?—another prescription. It was a very strong narcotic. Have you guessed it? Yes, Oxycontin. By now I had been on this medication twice before but not only was the dose never enough to really help but I was **entirely of the wrong mindset.** I was raging emotionally from the pain and the stress that so often accompanies trauma. Consequently I would take more than what was prescribed and run out way too soon, going through a couple of days of detoxification before I could get a new prescription. Both times I got off the medication abruptly. It was dreadful and took close to two weeks for it to get out of my system. In the meantime, the old suicide ideas were playing out in my mind. I had to find a better way to leave this dreadful existence. I had to *check out* somehow, or so I thought. But those bottles of pills never worked. I just wanted to be with God, not walking the earth and certainly not feeling the feelings. *Please, God, knock me out, bring me home with you. I'm tired.*

Going from the booze to a heavy narcotic tranquilizer like Klonopin, and then the Oxycontin was like going from the frying pan into the fire. I got sicker and sicker. Now even the pain pills were giving me no real relief. I heard Dr. A sigh again and again. What was he going to do with me? My life consisted of a progression of pain clinics, the fourth one in 1999, but the combination of drugs had affected me so severely that even they seemed to be giving up before we were barely started. Their approach, much like the last three clinics, was groups, modified exercise, and swimming. When I got down on a rubber pad on the floor, instead of following along with the exercises, I would just lie there not wanting to move. Surely they saw, as I did, that none of this was going to make any difference. In my mind I started planning a new method of suicide, one where I could die in nature with God and no one would find me or try to rescue me. I didn't want to be rescued; I wanted *out!*

The plan that was unfolding in my mind now was to somehow make my way to a wooded area in the mountains and valleys around Stony Creek in upper Dauphin County. We went there as kids when Mother and Father had a summer cottage. I wanted to find my way so deeply into the wilderness that no one could find me so I would starve and freeze to death. I was going to just disappear from everyone's lives. Susan was old enough by now to find her own life, and Don would find someone else. They didn't need me, surely, as much as I needed an escape. For a while I planned on getting a ticket to go to Lancaster County, further away, to carry this out. I even purchased it, but I later had a change of heart and took it back for a refund.

By 2001, Dr. A was passing me to other physicians for the Oxycontin prescriptions. I still indiscriminately took the little pink *wonder pills*—more like not so wonderful by now—always running out too soon. At one point I was going to a so-called pain clinic under Dr. W for the pills, but I heard the sighs and sensed, again, I was being given up on before we barely got started. Something that dug painfully into my awareness at this particular clinic was that a former classmate from the old Polyclinic Nursing School, Carol, worked there. I felt her accomplishment as a graduate and registered nurse, so wishing I too could have graduated.

Then, in August, I had complained so much to my family doctor—who can recall which of the many it was?—about chest pain that I was referred to a cardiologist for further studies. I must have sat in this specialist's office for over an hour, leafing through magazine after magazine and thinking, *Geesh, a person could die of a heart attack just waiting to be seen.* When I finally got into the examining room and talked with her, I complained of fainting while driving. Looking back I realize now they were not actual losses in consciousness but more like cognitive blanks—better known as *blackouts*.

The doctor was so worried about this she called for an ambulance. I tried to reason with her that my husband could come get me. Still, next thing I knew an EMT was starting an intravenous drip and injecting a substance called Narcan into my veins. She was taking it upon herself to strip all—and I mean *all*—the narcotics from my body. I convulsed and stopped breathing right there in her office. I was thrown into the ambulance and carted off to three different emergency rooms before they finally accepted me at the Medical Center in Hershey. It was here that a doctor attempted to get the ball rolling—to find a different solution for my knocked-out, drugged-out, decrepit existence. He recommended I go to a hospital *when I was ready* and get help getting off all the narcotics.

Two days later, under pressure from everyone, I had Don take me to the Holy Spirit Hospital Emergency Room so I could get this *help*, as they all called it. All I really wanted was for someone to cancel out this infernal ticket to hell I carried in my bruised subconscious. I sensed I was a lone actor on stage. No one felt what I was feeling. Nor did they know the sense of deep hurt and disappointment I had carried with me since that horrific fall into a stairwell. My child died that day, and I wanted her back, just like when I was ten years old and tried to will my doll baby to life. That is all I wanted, and of course the pain pills. But so far the pills only served to tease me like a cruel joke saying, "*Here, take this pill. It will cure you of all that ails you. You and your life are just a figment of someone's imagination, mostly your own. Stop trying to be someone you are not—stop trying to be human. You are only a broken piece of shit, so I want you to take this little bit of* encouragement *and hop back on the train we call* life."

Don took a personal day off work just to be with me as I attempted to collect myself. That afternoon we drove across the river to the hospital. A *danger* sign flashed in my head. What was I getting myself into? I knew the agony of detoxing from Oxycontin from two other times, and I certainly did not look forward to it. As we walked from the parking lot toward the emergency room, I said to Don, "Would you go on in and register me? I just need to stay out here and think a while." Well, if "think a while" means running willy-nilly across the parking lot and then crossing the Routes 11&15 bypass, well then I was *thinking*. But in reality, it was just me in escape mode again. I was lucky I didn't become road kill in the process. Obviously, I was not ready. I ended up at Dr. A's office in Wormleysburg a quarter mile away, where I called Don to come pick me up. If I recall exactly, I got home in time to put supper on the table. Life goes on.

I was determined I was going to somehow make my life work. I still wanted to be employed, so I applied for a local nursing home position, giving medications and doing treatments. I did what they called shadowing at the beginning, where I just followed another nurse around for a while. Then, when it was time to take over, I got so baffled that I could hardly function. It was that old feeling of *confusion* that had been with me over the years. But while I was here one day, I went to give medication to one of the residents in the courtyard where they were having a cookout when I heard a lilting Irish voice say, "Sylvia, is that you? Sylvia Hawthorn?" To my surprise, it was the mother of my old friend from elementary school, Robert Wentz.

I had wondered for years what happened to Robert, because he was a special friend. But we had lost track of each other in high school. Now I found out he was living down in Philadelphia. He had stayed there as a librarian at the University of Pennsylvania after he graduated. I was not surprised he became a bookworm. It suited him because he always shied away from the social scene. He would chase me home from school, but if my mother or father, or anyone, wanted to talk, he disappeared like a ghost. Now here he was hiding behind dusty old book shelves in the City of Brotherly Love, still riding his bicycle everywhere too. I loved this dear man as much as anyone can love an old friend, so I called him and asked him to come see us when he came up to visit his mother. But I did not expect what I was about to find out.

When I went to the train station to pick Robert up, I sat idling the car until a very tall, sickly older man with a gaunt yellow complexion shuffled toward me. He was no longer dashing at top speed like he used to. Of course not; we were grown adults now. All he had was a small duffel bag in his hand. It tore my heart out. He looked like a broken man. The next morning I took him to see his mother. It was then the reality of his situation in life came out.

I was told by the nurse on Mrs. Wentz's station that her son was not to be left alone in the room with her. The door had to be kept open during his visit and someone needed to be close by. Our *Bobby* was an alcoholic and had abused his mother. I was shocked and saddened by this information. How could the Robert I had loved as a child and a brilliant young man turn out so angry and an abuser of the one person who loved him dearly? I later found out from his live-in girlfriend about his struggle with booze—I was not surprised by the look of him—and what saddened me the most was that I learned he was dying of intestinal cancer.

I am a great believer that God puts certain people in our lives at just the right moment so that person in front of me now is there for a reason. This was just such an experience. I was soon to find out *why* Robert came back into my life and why I had to see this broken tragedy of a man. That was the last I saw of him. We spoke over the phone one more time when he expressed his desire to see me again, that maybe I could come to Philadelphia and we could take in a concert. I sensed he wanted to make up for lost time. But again as fate would have it, we both came to two different curves in our lives, curves that would this time separate us forever in this life.

By the winter of 2001 and January, February, and March of 2002, I was becoming more and more desperate. All I wanted was to die. Our daughter got married during this time, but I was so spaced out from the medication and the withdrawal into my own little hell that it felt—if I could feel anything—like a dream, a horror movie. I wanted to turn it off! Surely I would wake up and have a life again. Did I ever really have a life? Maybe it was all a dream. I clung to this single thought until April when, again, my life would change forever.

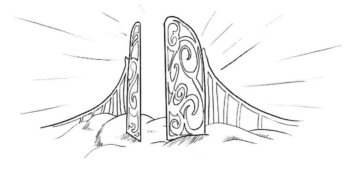

Part Two

Looking back, I see almost what seems like two lives: life before recovery and life after recovery. Life before recovery is vague; my husband recalls names, faces, and incidents where I draw a blank. I vaguely recall our daughter getting married. I was dopey and clumsy, nearly falling down the rise of the church sanctuary where the wedding was held. I do recall the lovely, pristine white angel on the seasonal evergreen that sat majestically nearby. I recall feeling like an overcooked dumpling because I had put on so much weight that I could barely squeeze into the lovely, deep red organza dress Susan had so tastefully picked out for me. I recall sitting about two-thirds of the way back from the front—probably as far as my husband wanted to take me for fear I would fall on my face. But there was one very important element missing in my life. It was *feelings*.

I knew I should have been feeling something or maybe even shedding a few tears. But all I could do was sit there like a lump or a piece of food that had fallen inadvertently onto the front of a clean blouse. I felt like one very big mistake sitting in a very sacred room, warmed by the soft glow of candles and resonating with the lilting sound of a flute. It was December of 2001, and little to my knowledge, I was standing at the brink of newness. My life was to soon evolve into a state I did not see coming. But in the moment, all I knew was emptiness and foreboding. *Have I died and are all these people here to mourn my death?*

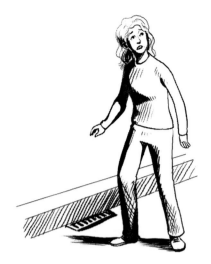

CHAPTER 5

The Walk to Find What Was Missing

On Friday, April 12, I had just bought a brand-new, expensive pair of sneakers. But I found myself sitting at home, as usual, drawing a blank. There seemed to be so much missing in my life that it didn't seem like a life at all. So, decked in my new shoes and a light jacket, I decided to go for a walk—a long one—looking for that something that was missing. I needed a sense of purpose, for one thing, but what kept me from finding it?

I walked from eight in the morning until five at night through housing developments and a shopping mall, through thickets, across highways and a stream. The only thing I got from the hike was very, very tired. I ended up back home in time for Don to get home and to get dinner on the table. Still, I found nothing of what I was looking for. Then, twenty-four hours later, I found it. I had a thorn embedded in my left palm from the thickets I had pushed aside during the walk. Now I at least knew what was missing— feelings! Four days later, on April 16, 2002, I was only a day short of getting my medication, but this time was different. I had Don once again take me to that hospital, but this time I went in. I was ready.

Detoxification is a big word but not as big as the feelings and the heightened senses a person goes through in the process. Not only did they take my Oxycontin from me—I didn't have any anyway—but they took the Klonopin too. Then they stuck me in a room with nothing but a mattress on the floor, a sink, and some equipment on the wall. When I complained of pain that first day, they did something I sorely regretted afterward. They gave me a Motrin, just what I *didn't* need on top of a nervous, ulcerated stomach from my years of drinking. And with my heightened senses, even the vinyl tubing attached to suction on the wall of that little hellish room made me throw up. I vomited my guts out and was nauseated for the next whole week, losing twelve pounds in the process. I was in that emergency room for four days, unable to sleep for all the noise and confusion, and I felt like death warmed over. Had someone turned me inside out and strewn me out for the buzzards?

On the third day, right after being moved from the confines of that little crash pad, Don came to see me with some sad news: my friend, Robert, had died of his alcoholism and cancer. After this everything became a blur. What was going to happen to me? Was the whole world falling apart? Mine was, I was certain. I remembered a meditation the biofeedback therapist, Dr. Fink[iv], had done with me in the past year, so I lay there in my state of anguish going into a self-made trance.

I pictured myself on an escalator going down, down, down … into a room filled with dusty leather-bound books on all sides. I had created this room. Down in this sacred spot, I felt the presence of Christ. For the longest time I talked with this wonderful, sensitive man, telling him of all the years I had struggled and asking him to come with me on the rest of my journey. I needed him, his compassion, and his love. Finally, after four days, I was moved to a bed on the fourth floor in a lonely room at the end of a long hall with just a call bell, a TV set, and a crucifix on the wall. Not too many people came in, except the volunteers with magazines, quiet nuns with cheerful smiles, and various doctors and nurses. I recall one doctor in particular I will call Dr. H because I recognized him later at an AA meeting.

Dr. H visited me on Sunday morning, and more than anyone else, he seemed to reach out to me. I didn't know why at the time, but I did take the opportunity to ask him, "Do you think this thorn will come out?" I showed him the palm of my left hand. "Oh, yes, Mrs. Deppen, it will work its way out." With that and another pleasant smile, he left. But the thorn never came out. I was glad because to me, that thorn represented my conviction to live again, to get my life together and not look back. I became willing to do whatever it took.

Our daughter and new son-in-law came in that day too and brought a diary I had asked them to get for me. I was having all these thoughts and feelings rush back into my mind and body, and I needed to write things down. This was not just some little cardboard notebook they brought me; it was bound in dark brown leather, and it smelled so refreshing to my struggling, heightened senses and lurching stomach. As I took in one long whiff of the fragrant leather, I worked my fingers over its smooth, cool, dark surface. My first entry shows how fixed my thinking was on our daughter at the time as I began to remember what had been behind the cloud of the drugs:

> Monday April 22, 2002
>
> Dear Susan, my precious daughter,
> Last night, standing naked in the shower tub here at the hospital, I recalled the fear you had as a child with that big drain in our bathtub at home. You were so small, and when I took the stopper out, I think you were sure you were going down the drain. What is the saying? "Don't throw the baby out with the bath water"?
> Yeah.
> Susan, this last week has been, I believe, one of the most difficult in my life—detoxification. Yes, it will take gumption for me to get up and go again. I have been so long shadowed by medicine. It's why I missed you growing up!

Later that day I wrote this:

> Monday evening, April 22, still
>
> Boy, what a long day getting here to Marworth Treatment Center. I think they call it "living sober". It is the twelve-step program used by Alcoholics Anonymous and Narcotics Anonymous.

> Dad [Don] drove 260 miles to get me here. Of course
> Buddy [our dog] came along for the company—and for
> the doggy bag from Perkins Pancakes. The food was
> good—real good—to me. We got here to Marworth, near
> Scranton, and it was so cold. But the trees were budding
> and sprouting. It was snowing by the time we arrived.

I had never been in a rehab, and I remember the trip like it was yesterday. Don took me in my little red Chevy Cavalier. Buddy, our faithful beagle, long-haired dachshund, lay patiently in the backseat as we drove the nearly three hundred miles to Waverly, Pennsylvania, where Marworth Treatment Center is located. I stared out the window at the bleak countryside passing beside us as I struggled to straighten my depleted body. This felt like the end of my life—surely I was dying. Surely I would not wake up tomorrow. Or maybe this was all just a bad dream and I would wake up in my bed at home in the city where I lived so many years ago, before the nightmare began. But now, in the moment, my life felt like a cold, desolate wilderness, and I was waiting for the end.

Yes, it was one very long day. But it was at just this point, too, that another light began to shine into the darkness. My life *was* changing. I could feel it as my fingers worked over the smooth leather of the diary that night and I drifted into the first short but solid sleep since it all began five days before.

The rehab was built in and around the childhood estate of Mary Worthington, the wife of the late Pennsylvania governor William Scranton, and had been converted, in her memory, into a drug and alcohol rehabilitation center run by Geisinger Medical Center in Danville. It was a large stone house with various wings and extensions built onto it to accommodate the increasing population of addicts and alcoholics, many of them medical professionals and pharmacists, coming to their door. On the evening I arrived in late April, there was a light, damp snowfall. The first thing they did was take all of my luggage, returning just the bare necessities. Don stayed with me only a short time. We kissed, and that was the last we even talked for three days. It was the first time in our twenty-four years of marriage we did not talk at least once a day. Now all I had was a calling card and the hopes I would soon talk to him again. I felt estranged and frightened.

I was admitted to the detox area, where they kept me sedated on Phenobarbital for the withdrawal symptoms—"good shit," they called it. I was weighed, interviewed, and examined by a physician's assistant and a psychiatrist. I was surprised they did not fingerprint me with the full extent of their inquiry. For the first two days, I was assigned a buddy, a young woman who had already been there two months, to help guide me down a very long hall to the cafeteria, dining room, and various meeting rooms.

One room, built off the main house, had a huge picture window—floor to ceiling—and once when we were having a meeting there, a doe and her fawn came up and grazed silently. This room was appropriately named "The God Room." At meal time everyone lined up outside the cafeteria and roll call was taken. I don't know where they expected me to go. There was nothing but a stone wall, fields, barren country road, and forest surrounding the estate. I struggled, weak from the detox and years of inactivity, to get one foot in front of the other without falling on my face. I recalled a record we listened to as children, "The Little Engine that Could," and said to myself over and over, "I gotta make it, gotta make it, gotta make it …"

The primary message was, "*Step One: We admitted we were powerless over [something]—that our lives had become unmanageable.*" The obvious message everyone was sharing, with little reservation, was their various addictions. They called this their "drug of choice." I sensed many of the patients had been drinking and using street drugs. The drinking rang a bell, but the street drug thing was something new to me. Regardless, I got the message: Drugs and alcohol can steal your soul. They got that right. They "steal your soul", I realized later, when you have no other means of finding peace and tranquility. All of us look at various times in our life for relief from the mad, mad world or as in my case, relief from pain.

I truly wondered what they expected me to do for this pain I had carried around for forty-eight years. Doesn't someone have a bag a tricks they can reach into and relieve me of the agony? Surely the revelation of my life when I realized how I had fallen nearly to my death and the state of affairs in my face and neck would give one of these professionals an idea of how best to help me. "Surely, *surely*," as the Psalm goes, "*goodness and mercy shall follow me for all the days of my life.*" Just who were "*Goodness*" and "*Mercy*"? Were they characters from *Pilgrim's Progress?* I felt like I had to click my heels, my ruby slippers, and repeat the words, "I want to go home … I want to go home …"

I lay awake through the better part of most nights. I was beginning to think full nights of sleep were a thing of the past. One of those nights, right after being moved from detox into a regular room with just one roommate, I got up and strolled to the women's lounge across the hall. When I walked in, I saw the twelve steps of recovery printed on scrolls to either side of the room. One whole outside wall was another massive picture window looking out into a wooded area. I felt like I had a view of what heaven must look like. Then I gravitated to the scroll on my far left marked, "Step 6: *We were entirely ready for God to remove all these defects of character.*" I prayed quietly, "God, I need you to take away my defective borderline personality. Please just take this from me."

As a licensed nurse, I was to stay for three months, but when they took me off the Phenobarbital, they did it too quickly, and it was like someone pushed the replay button. The old suicide tapes reran in my head. I shared this with a nurse, and they scheduled me for a quick discharge. I was only at Marworth for a little over a week when they sent me home. And just like at Phil Haven, I had a prescription for the twelve steps of Alcoholics Anonymous or Narcotics Anonymous in my pocket. This time I knew I had to keep going to meetings. I was told to do ninety meetings in ninety days. However, this time I was gifted with enough desperation that it would stick.

I will never forget the weekend before leaving they showed a movie, *Field of Dreams,* with Kevin Costner. Then I knew I would dream again. I knew there was some hope for me in these rooms of recovery. I may not have been a street drug addict or the skid row bum lying in a gutter, but I was someone who needed her own personal story of recovery and a voice to be heard by others. In turn I needed to hear theirs too because even though the details may have been different, it was basically the same— looking for comfort in the bottom of a gin bottle or from countless pills. I was finding that person in myself that I had been searching for. And I actually liked her.

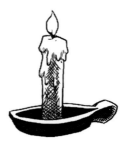

HAPPY, HEALTHY, AND *HOLY* …

*"God would be mocked if any of His creations
lacked holiness. The creation is whole, and
the mark of wholeness is holiness."*[v]

It was May of 2002, and after twenty-seven psych admissions, six suicide attempts, eleven surgeries—you would think I would be *fixed* by now—and hundreds of hours over twenty-one years in Dr. A's cozy little crash pad and talk tank, I came home from rehab ready to face life on life's terms. I was still racked with pain and spasms, but now I had a lot more to think about: meetings, getting a sponsor, doing the steps, and still just having a life, a husband, and a family that still, somehow, loved me. Our daughter was married and living in Middletown, but I could barely remember the wedding. I am certainly not proud of the lack of clarity in my memory, but I am proud my daughter turned out so beautifully in spite of my absence in her life. Fortunately, she took on a lot of her dad's character traits. Now I had to somehow find a way to make my life work, even though the old pain issues still barked at the back door.

One night Don attended family night with me at the hospital where I was signed up for their intensive drug and alcohol program. We watched the movie *When a Man Loves a Woman* with Andy Garcia and Meg Ryan. It felt like someone was throwing all my bad behaviors over those drinking years back in my face, like it was all just happening. We drove home in silence, and as we crossed the bridge over the Susquehanna River, one of the old suicide tapes of me jumping flashed into my weary mind. The misery was still upon me. I *had* to find a way to deal with it that I could live without suffering, but how?

It was May 30 and Memorial Day weekend. I was cleaning out the back of my car and found a set of tapes, copies, given to me by the same biofeedback therapist, Dr. Fink, who had given me the escalator meditation I had used successfully in the emergency room. I had thrown the tapes there because at the time all I wanted was *my* pills, the Oxy and Klonopin. But now I had nothing but the psych meds. What could I lose? I decided I'd try them. I took them into the house and began listening and listening and listening ... I listened hour after hour, sometimes six and seven hours a day, when I wasn't at meetings. The voice of Shinzen Young and *Break through Pain* became so familiar my day was not complete without hearing him. This is when it all began for me—a complete house cleaning and change in my thinking.

By June I started to feel that a kind of space was opening up inside me, a place so familiar and yet so strange. I had to go to the dictionary and look up one word: *nirvana*. I never knew such a place existed, where I was comfortable and free of suffering. All the years I had read of heaven in the Bible and heard pastors and Sunday school teachers talk of this marvelous place we go when we lead good lives and die. There it was, right in my own living room. Shinzen Young was telling me, just like he was sitting across from me, "Sylvia, if you have severe physical and emotional pain, you might have to become like a monk in a monastery and learn to meditate for relief." And instead of fleeing the pain, I was to move through it; what a novel idea.

Day after day I went on listening until the two tapes wore out and I had to order my own set. They wore out again, so I ordered more. I listened so much that eventually they were in my head. I could do them anywhere, anytime, even with my eyes open driving a car. By July and August I realized what was happening. I was *healing*, not from the outside-in like the pills and therapy were supposed to do, but instead from the inside-out, where it counted. I would go for little walks between half-hour sessions, and I noticed what I called little "pleasure bubbles" rising to my conscious mind. They were fleeting memories of when I was yet five years old—before the trauma—and a happy child. They would rise and quickly *pop!* But oh, what a gift it was to have the child back in my life. I could see her standing next to me, dressed in her little plaid dress with the white Peter Pan collar, the same dress I wore when I fell into that infamous stairwell. It was so magical that one day I bought a little Harry Houdini bear on display at the post office. I keep him on hand for my meditation groups today at the hospital. Yes, I was finally healing, and the pain, instead of being my curse, became my *gift*. It's hard to imagine but true.

THE *MAGIC* OF MIND TRAINING

The mind or brain is a powerful organ. Just think for a moment what it can do. Consider the situation where there is a horrendous accident and a mother watches as her child is trapped under a car. With but the flick of a switch—quickly!—in her brain, she reaches out and with all of her 120 or 130 pounds lifts that huge vehicle, thus freeing the child she so loves. Think, too, that the mind holds data from years and years of a person's life. Memories from twenty, thirty, forty, and even fifty or more years ago stream into the conscious mind. The data released can be as if the events in that time of life are just happening: tastes, smells, and feelings come to mind as fresh as the day and the moment they occurred.

Yes, the mind is a powerful entity, where tiny cells connect in intricate, revealing sequences, allowing us to relive so much. All the while, the autonomic system keeps a myriad of organs functioning rhythmically: the breath, the heartbeat, the stomach, intestines, and other vital organs. But above all, it gives us control of what is happening to and around us, so we interpret it all and can literally decide what to do with the information streaming through to us. When we are warm, cozy, tired, and well fed, we can drift into a night of restful sleep and God/Spirit-induced dreams. The same goes for a stressful situation.

When we are faced with a stressful and/or painful situation, we can either tell ourselves, "This is an impossible situation and I don't believe it can be rectified." Or "I have been in a tight situation before and it has been okay. I can do this!" What we tell ourselves is often what can make or break a situation. It took diligent hours of listening to suggested thoughts in *Break through Pain* to change my own perception and life outcome. I had to turn nearly a lifetime of negative, reactive thinking into livable thought patterns, thus changing my own brain waves. There is literally a *symphony*[vi] going on in our heads, and we can either be the conductors or let others tell us how we should look, sense, feel, and be. My, what power we truly have over our lives.

MIRACLES

Still Waters Run Deep

In August of 2002, something else happened to put the cap on healing for me. Dr. Fink had also given me the name of a meditation teacher, Lois Dunnevant, and she gave classes in meditation at a place called Almateracom. This was a center where they had whole rooms with cushions and little altars and candles for meditating. I will never forget the evening I went for her class.

It was in a big room with chairs sitting around in a semicircle. Lois was a petite little lady with a gentle voice. To begin the class, she wrote with blue dry erase marker on the board, "Still waters run deep." She was then suddenly called to go out of the room for a phone call. When she came back in, we all looked with amazement at the words she had written on the board. Something caused the last few words to run to the bottom of the board. "Wow," she said. "Still waters really do run deep."

She also put a diagram on the board of the Jungian Pyramid that demonstrated how meditation affects our access to the different levels of the mind: the conscious mind, where the ego reigns; the personal subconscious, where our dreams speak to us of our gifts and how to use them; and the universal subconscious, where our prayers reach others and theirs reach us, with the Ground Buddha, or Holy Spirit, down at the bottom feeding us from the *Spirit World*. I learned that *that* Spirit was the reason for meditation, and by accessing it, I could learn a whole slew of information not just about myself and my past but about others in my life. This is the reason for meditation: to heal all life.

I was indeed healing in leaps and bounds. On the way out that evening, I boroughed a set of tapes in their library called "Healing the Unhealed Healer." They were eight sessions with Dr. Kenneth Wapnick of the Foundation for Inner Peace and *The Course in Miracles*. I reasoned, *Well, I am a healthcare professional, supposedly, and I could use some more healing.* I mean, I was on a roll now. So I took those eight tapes home with me and on vacation to the Outer Banks in September. I must have listened to the eight tapes three times, but I was so frustrated trying to figure out what this man was trying to say that as soon as we got home, I went to take them back to Almateracom. But before I got to the door, the message hit me like a bolt of lightning. I had to go back to the car and start listening all over. So much more healing poured over me because I realized how much forgiving I had to do. Resentments of my mother were piled deeply in every direction.

In November of 2002, I was taking a Sunday-afternoon nap when I had a familiar dream. It was one of those dreams you've had before where you think there must be a message, but what is it? In the dream I was knocking on a row of doors, but this time just before I woke up, the doors began opening! I was left with this thought, finally, that opportunities were coming and I would see there was real purpose for my being on this earth. I sat for a moment, absorbing the meaning of the dream, and then I took off for a 4:00 pm AA meeting. At that meeting a man we all knew as Jim D. shared that his mother had just died and he was in mourning. It occurred to me that my mother had died eight years before and I never mourned her passing. How could I? She was rushed away and cremated so quickly I never got to say good-bye. I was too numb at the time anyway.

I had listened to a lot of Carolyn Myss' work. She is known especially for her skills as a medical intuitive and her "Sacred Contracts" and with the chakras in a work called, *The Science of Medical Intuition* along with Dr. Norman Sheely.[vii] She taught me that if I want closure with someone who has passed on, I just need to light a candle and talk to that person. That evening, alone in my meditation area of the house, I lit a candle to talk to

Mother. But as soon as I lit it, it went out! All I could think was, *Okay, Mother, I know you don't want to talk; you never did.* That evening I was on the way to my precious Wednesday-night women's AA meeting when I heard the words loud and clear, *You don't have to light a candle to talk to me, Sylvia.* It was definitely my mother, and from then on I felt her dynamic presence in my life, guiding me and allowing things to happen for me.

I felt her presence another time too. It was early one morning, which is always the best time to meditate for me, and I was just finishing up a forty-five-minute Stephen Levine meditation when suddenly near the end I heard the words, "Put your head on my shoulder." For about ten minutes I could smell my mother's apron, like I was a small child in her arms. All I could think afterward was, *What a blessing.* She really was with me, wasn't she? It didn't take some psychic or magic trick or even a candle. She was simply there for me. And best of all, she really did want to talk. I have wondered why I don't get that kind of closure with my father, but I came to realize I *am* my father. I have so many of his character traits that I am a living, breathing, female version of him.

> *Wheel going around and around, clicking, spinning, driving*
> *me further into life, away from, toward. Where have I*
> *begun, where have I been, where am I going? I just keep*
> *pedaling, around and around ... I saw what I saw, I see*
> *what I see, I will see what there is to see. Oh, wheel going*
> *around and around, clicking, spinning, driving me further,*
> *further, further ... When I stop, nobody knows; where I*
> *stop I know not either. I just am, I just am, I ... just ... am.*
> *I ... am ... I am ... I ... I ... I ... am ... am ... am ...*

So now I had my meetings, my meditation, and my *Course in Miracles.* All of this was working together for a healing I barely saw coming. In the meantime, my bicycle had sat collecting dust in the garage. I had been so rundown and sick that I had not gone for a ride—my favorite mode of transportation—for years. I finally was able to get that beautiful, ten-speed Raleigh out, dust it off, get the tires fixed, and off I went. It occurred to me that if I worked hard at riding, maybe—just maybe—someday I could ride from *Pennsylvania* to Florida instead of from South Carolina like I did in the '70s. This has become a large part of my dream today, to ride the over two thousand miles to Naples, Florida. My new dream took shape; *I* got in shape too. After all, Ed Mood from the Bicycle Club back then had done it at the ripe old age of seventy-four. Why shouldn't I?

Starting up again was rough. I didn't realize how much muscle mass I had lost from lying around. And that first summer, 2003, I had three flat tires. When I went to the bike shop the third time to pick it up, Ted, the bike shop owner, asked me, "Where are you riding your bicycle that you keep having flats?" I replied, "Well, off to the side out of the way of traffic." Then he told me, "Sylvia, get back into the traffic. All the nails and screws and glass fly onto the side. That's why you are having all these flats."

I had to get up my courage to ride with the cars. After having been hit from behind—in the dark—back in 1974, I keep a watchful eye on what is coming up behind me. But now, I was really back into the flow and working up the courage I needed in my life. Sure, people get hit on their bikes all the time, but as someone once told me, a life lived in fear is not much fun. And look at it this way: so what if I get wiped out, *what a way to go …*

From the time I rode as a child on an old American-made, one speed, brakes-in-the-pedals bicycle, I have loved riding. It is a way to keep the *chi* flowing and my chakras unblocked. *That* is why I ride today at the ripe young age of sixty-four. And now, with all the healing in my life and in spite of my continuing pain issues, I want to live until I am a hundred, maybe longer. I found early in recovery that my pain had become a gift, and with that gift came renewed energy. Meditation had actually turned the blocked, stagnant pain into a brand-new source of energy. Now I also felt like I had something to contribute to this life. What I went through was certainly very, very difficult. But it made me who I am today, and that's okay.

The year after I came into recovery, 2003, a neurosurgeon removed clusters of spurs off my neck and I could turn my head freely again. I could finally get rid of the cervical collar I had been wearing for over a year. And the ice packs for spasms were long gone by now. Also in June of that year I began doing volunteer work for the Drug and Alcohol Intensive Outpatient Program I had just completed at the hospital . Every few weeks I took music and meditations to their patients, offering the same help I got from meditation and prayer . This keeps it fresh for me too.

The eleventh step is a kind of prayer to find *"God's will for us and the power to carry it out."* I was finally realizing it was not God making me suffer all those years; it was me. And through the meditation—not the medication—the really deep connection with Spirit, I was letting go of my fixation on the pain and how much it was causing me to suffer. All this was in exchange for a renewed life force.

Answers and inspirations began pouring into my conscious mind. I never dreamed of going on a cruise to Alaska, but we did in August for our twenty-fifth wedding anniversary. I deliberately got fitted with contact lenses to add to the romance of the voyage, but Don never even noticed. He was too busy taking pictures and delighting in the gourmet buffets. He apologized later, but I didn't care; I was just glad I could be with him—I mean totally with him—and no longer preoccupied with suffering. Sometime later I noticed Don looking at me, shaking his head, and laughing. I had seen him do this before, so I asked him what he was laughing at. Chuckling, he replied, "I just don't know you anymore, Sylvia." And I knew he meant it in a good way.

Now, as part of being the enlightened new person I had become, and with a background in *A Course in Miracles*, I easily forgave a lot in my life. I forgave the people in my past as well as everyone and everything in the present. I forgave myself, too, for having essentially failed at nursing. But that did not mean I wouldn't try nursing again. When someone is ingrained with an idea of who they are at an early age, like five, it is extremely difficult to break that vision, especially since it is a profitable one. I now at least understood that even though healthcare givers are considered healers, only the individual, the patient, can truly heal him or herself from within. I still took the psychotropic medications and went for counseling—still do—because all that helped. But it was up to me to let go of the past and my ideas of who I thought I was.

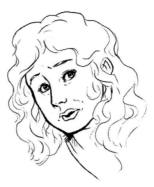

CHAPTER 6

Happy, Healthy, and Whole

I now had two major tasks in front of me: the steps of recovery and getting back to work. In other words, I had to meet life on life's terms. I was raised to believe in hard work. But was I going to be able to work? I was ready to give it my best effort. In the first year of recovery, I took a nursing refresher course. I had sponsors, good ones, in recovery, and I worked the steps even though I never had a sponsor who really insisted on it. I would just quietly work on step one, then two, then three in my head and then write what was happening. Recovery was about experience, strength, and hope; or, *what it was like* (before recovery), *what happened* (how my recovery came about), and *what it was like now* (how recovery affected my life).

Some people think enlightenment is something only the Buddha or some guru can achieve. But between May 30 and June 30, 2002, I found enlightenment. By June, I felt something change deep inside me. It was like a big space opened up in me, and it was here where I was very, very, *very* comfortable. Some days, when I was feeling the worst, I had difficulty tuning into the sessions. But it was these days that my practice really took hold. The *Circulation of Awareness, Real Estate of Your Pain, Working with Space,* and *Expanding and Contracting with the Breath*[viii] stayed with me. I didn't need the tapes all the time. Then the next day I would go back to the tapes. Gifted with desperation, I worked at this so diligently. My husband laughed at me but only because he was starting to relax after so many years of worry. In the mornings, when he was ready to go to work, I would come out of the back room where I meditated and kiss him good-bye. Then, at five o'clock when he came home, I would once again come out of *my* room and greet him with a kiss. He did not mind the time I was spending meditating because, of anyone, he realized the most that I was doing what I needed to do for myself.

Yes, I was becoming an enlightened person. I knew too that once this happened I could never be *un*-enlightened. I would have good days and bad days—that comes with being human. But I could never be that miserable, hopeless person I had been before. And after only a month of this splendid relief from suffering, *I decided, if it took my last breath on earth, I would teach one other person to meditate and find peace and comfort.* I felt no one could put a price tag on this, and I realized that God's will was not that I, or anyone, should suffer; that is our incorrect thinking. Suffering comes of obsessive thinking or focusing so much on the pain that we miss the pleasure. In fact, I found out pain and pleasure are on opposite sides of the same coin. If I throw away the pain, I am no doubt throwing away pleasure too. Something else happened from this process.

As a result of the meditation, I experienced a phenomenon called *purification* (i.e., as the spiritual and psychological blockages in me became broken up, my spirit was freed). This allows me access to the Spirit World. I have never been so aware of being surrounded by the spirits of my ancestors and of those who were there for me before I was born. I am vitally aware too that they await me in the next life. I can talk freely with them and am often aware of messages they have for me. Am I a psychic? No, not really. I cannot name these spirits because in the other life, there are no names, just feelings. And they are the most wonderful, freeing feelings I have ever experienced. I am delighted to tell you that you can find a state of purification too. Go for it. Practice meditation every free moment you get—especially mornings, after a night of good sleep. The Spirit World wants you to know they are always there for you.

Betty Eadie, an LPN like myself and the mother of eight children, experienced death in a hospital after a hysterectomy, and she had this to say about spirit communication:

They communicated much more rapidly and completely, in a manner they referred to as "pure knowledge." The closest word in English we would have to define it is telepathy, but even that doesn't describe the full process. I felt their emotions and intents. I felt their love.[ix]

From the *Course in Miracles* I learned also that my task on this earth was to help others learn there is no final judgment on our souls, no sin, no guilt, and no separation or fall from grace as portrayed in the Bible; that comes of fear-based thinking. Without fear, a lot in this life would change, including all sickness. No matter what the affliction, it would disappear without fear. Fear does manifest in very real symptoms that make us *think* we are ill when in truth we are whole beings deceived by our own, often-subconscious, guilt and trepidation—all instruments of the ego. Without these, we are well and happy human beings.

This and only this is what is real. We are all entitled to be happy, healthy, whole, *and* holy.

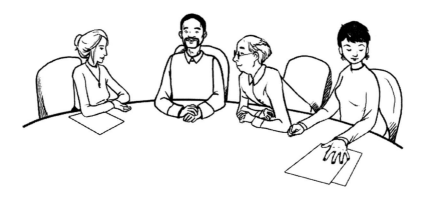

CHAPTER 7

Life on Life's Terms

My first two years of recovery were about nothing *but* recovery. I began writing my way into and through the steps regularly. Then, when I began the process of going back to work, I began writing regularly just about life on life's terms as it pertained to my recovery. Those early years were devoted to my *"journey inward"* (i.e., what was going on inside me). Later, after going back to work, it became my *"journey outward"* (i.e., how what was inside me related to what was going on outside). This way I could have an ongoing dialogue with *Spirit*, now my inner source of strength and knowledge, as well as a conversation with life in general, my source of learning, and participating in my husband's and family's lives.

One thing is for sure: while going to work complicated the process a bit, it also made it more interesting. As long as I was living the steps, I knew now my life would be okay.

STEP 1: "WE ADMITTED WE WERE POWERLESS OVER ALCOHOL/DRUGS/ *PAIN*—THAT OUR LIVES HAD BECOME UNMANAGEABLE."

I thoroughly understood how powerless I had been over the pills, mostly because they never helped completely. I needed a new mindset too. The

Klonopin depressed me, and I became so clumsy I was falling all over the place. The twenty milligrams of Oxycontin barely took the edge off the spinal pain. I was trying to obliterate all the pain, and that was just not going to happen, not with the kind of bizarre, distorted, and negative thinking that went on in my scruffy little head. After all, I later realized a person has to have *some* pain just to feel alive. The meetings help me see that everyone has pain in some aspect of their bodies and lives. Why should I be exempt?

For over the eight years of my early recovery, I said the words, "I'm Sylvia, and I am an alcoholic." I said it so many times I believed it. I had to—for one thing the state of Pennsylvania put restrictions on my nursing license so I had to do meetings at least twice a week. That did not matter to me so much because I liked the rigors of going to meetings. I trudged and labored through those ninety meetings in ninety days because I was so weak at first. But it was in the ninth year of recovery that things changed.

I had been powerless those years of heavy drinking, but what I was really powerless over was the pain. I stopped drinking when I almost hit a woman while I was driving drunk. But I thoroughly believe what was really behind my giving up the drink was that every time I drank, the ensuing detoxification process made my pain ten times worse—so I kept drinking! And when the psychiatrist started me on the Klonopin, well, that was just a nasty drug meant to remedy the wild thinking. The Oxycontin might have helped but no one ever tried to find a dose that actually helped. It is just as well, though, because by being forced to come off of it, I found the true power of positive, re-adjusted thinking. As a result of taking too much for almost five years, I would run out too soon, going through a day or two of withdrawal—understandably the pain was much worse—and then start all over, trying to treat the pain with a dose that did not work and a mindset that was frantic! It was a mad, *mad* life, chasing comfort, when all the while out of control thinking had been the real culprit.

In 2007, I had had my neck fused at two levels to help stop the spasms. It was wonderful for six months. But I had been warned by Dr. Fink that spinal surgery of any kind could create new problems. Well, guess what? It did. I was still relieved of those spasms, but now my upper back that had caused so much chest pain over the years started giving me spinal pain too—an old affliction gone awry. After seven months of taking constant doses of Vicodin—yes, I went back to some pain medication—my doctor said he feared all the acetaminophen or Tylenol, a major component of this medication, might cause liver failure. The doctor's wife had a liver transplant for this reason. He insisted, "I cannot give you anything but Oxycontin." I respected him for this decision, but I was taken back by the suggestion. I just did not want to go back to that merry-go-round.

I stewed over this for months, but out of agony, I finally gave in. Again, it just kind of teased me, but this time I was at least given a supplement of an instant-release kind of morphine known as oxycodone. This was new to me, and it actually helped. Plus, I realized that combined with my new, enlightened, and more-relaxed mindset, it actually was helping—a little. At the time I was getting very, very frustrated and angry with my physician for not helping me get closure with this new version of an old affliction. Still, in my mind I wanted someone to try to *fix it*. I wanted an MRI, and I wanted to see the neurosurgeon who had taken the spurs off my neck in 2003, thinking maybe it was just more spurs causing it. But he kept ordering the wrong tests! I started to get so angry at him, but having jumped from physician to physician before recovery, I did not want to get a new doctor.

Finally, two years later I found a new physician and finally got the necessary testing. But to my dismay, the orthopedic physician told me, "If we operate, Sylvia, we could create even more problems." It helps tremendously that I have finally been able to let go of the anger that came of all this conflict. The doctor also adjusted my pain medication to where I actually had the kind of relief I needed. As I look back at those years, I see that, first, *anxiety* popped up and bit me in the butt. (The anxiety was from many, many years of suffering.) And second, the *anger* made things even worse. (The anger was generalized but mostly pointed to just negative thinking.) These two factors influence how I tolerate or do not tolerate pain. But still, a part of me—deep down—hated being back on Oxycontin.

For so many years the rooms of recovery were telling me, Oxycontin is a bad drug; *get off the drug!* This is why I resisted so being put back on it. Finally, my new physician sat me down for a heart-to-heart talk. His words to me were, "Sylvia, you are in a lot of pain. I mean, just look at your past. People with this kind of pain need and benefit from pain medicine. Stop fighting it!" And guess what? I stopped fighting it. Now I get even more help from it. It is that resistance that created more suffering. As a scholar of

Shinzen Young's *Break through Pain*, why didn't I think of that? Something else changed in my recovery over this period.

Yes, I had said, *"I'm an alcoholic,"* so many times, I believed it. But when I came into recovery, I had not drunk for eight years. And with *my* pain—I have to own this kind of monster in me that has so often reared its ugly head—I have been seeking out comfort foods, like macaroni and cheese, a pint of ice cream at one sitting, or can after can of Bush's baked beans. Plus the psych meds I have been on cause high cholesterol. This bothered me. I did not want to have a heart attack after recovering from years of being sick. I understood that a glass of wine in the evening, perhaps with a meal or during a happy hour, helps to promote longevity. I wanted to live a long time, if I could. What a change from trying to do myself in all those times.

So I quietly started having one glass of wine right before bed. I allowed myself no more than this. Eventually I told Don what I was doing, and although he was skeptical at first, he saw too that it was not affecting my recovery. I have held off from telling any of my cohorts in AA about this, not wanting to cause a relapse in any of them. After all, many of them are brittle alcoholics. Today Don is looking at retirement next year, so whenever we get a chance, we have our own little happy hour. This bothered me at first because I was still going to AA meetings. But now I realize I am *still sober*—neither the Oxycontin nor the alcohol have caused me to lose objectivity. I simply cannot *self-medicate* with alcohol. Nor can I take any more than the prescribed dose of Oxycontin. If I do—well for one thing, I would run out again too soon. But for another, I know I am not taking time for mindfulness, reading, and meditation—all instruments of my sanity and continued health.

I have to pinch myself sometimes and ask, "Is this still you, Sylvia?" But yes, it is me. Mother and Father were right; I'm *not* an alcoholic. I just enjoy and need the meetings, so now I go to Chronic Pain Anonymous instead of Alcoholics Anonymous. They keep me grounded. That is why I use the twelve steps today for powerlessness over pain. A person can keep seeking more and more surgery over the years, often putting him or herself in harm's way by doing so. Surgery has all kinds of risks. Yes, death is one. But the danger of creating more havoc in the body, especially that created by spinal surgery, poses some of the worst after-effects. I am proof of that. There are plenty of others, I'm sure, who can attest to this too.

If you plan on looking for this kind of remedy, you'd best ground yourself spiritually and mindfully first. It will be like a kind of insurance plan. Depending entirely on the surgery is risky. However, this kind of commitment takes time and patience, something that seems in short supply these days. Have you noticed lately that a moment of silence is only ten or twenty seconds? And that is only if you are lucky? I strive not to short myself just because people around me are shorting themselves.

STEP 2: "WE CAME TO BELIEVE THAT A POWER GREATER THAN OURSELVES COULD RESTORE US TO SANITY."

My work with the second step started when I went to a meeting at the recovery clubhouse on South Nineteenth Street in Harrisburg. I don't know why it happened there. It just kind of jumped off the chart on the wall.

My life had definitely been insane. I had been in that revolving door to the psych ward over two dozen times in the twenty-one years I had been with Dr. A. My first counselor in recovery was a man I adored—Dr. Ramirez—but after a while I asked for a woman counselor because he reminded me too much of growing up with a dominant brother. He took it well, even laughed when I told him. I needed someone who let me do my own thinking. Dr. Ramirez, however, was the person who lifted my borderline personality diagnosis, the diagnosis Dr. A took a whole weekend to come up with because he said, "You just do not fit any one diagnosis very well." I can only assume my suicidal behavior was equated with people who have this diagnosis and cut themselves. I didn't mind giving up that title. Who wants a diagnosis at all if they don't need one? In fact, Dr. Ramirez said he thought I probably never did deserve the handle, which was given to me only for the purpose of getting Social Security Disability.

So to put it clearly, I was not insane. That is, I was no more insane than anyone else around me. I learned from *The Course in Miracles* that to be in this illusive world is to be insane because it was all just that—an illusion. The only sane part of life is the miracles that come of simply loving and being loved, and forgiving and being forgiven. Before latching onto the course and hearing my Aunt Aileen speak of it, I thought to myself, *Even if there is such a thing as a* miracle, *I would not deserve one.* Boy was I wrong, because I found out later miracles are going on all the time—around me and everybody.

My new counselor, Kathy Russell, was a lovely lady in her fifties who was also in recovery. Kathy became a close and dependable confidante. She always gave me a full hour, during which time I would practically talk her ear off. She introduced me to another woman, Louise Hay, and her book *You Can Heal Your Life.* Louise Hay taught me that there is not any part of our bodies—any symptom or collection of symptoms—that cannot be healed through positive affirmation and turning our thoughts around to get a different view of life. I use this kind of practice to stop the spasms in my body today with these words, either spoken out loud or to myself: *"I release, relax, and let go. I am safe."* It really works. Wonder of wonders, something besides pills actually does more than anything ever did—not the ice packs, the hot pads, the cervical collar, nor especially the narcotic tranquilizer.

STEP 3: "WE MADE A DECISION TO TURN OUR WILL AND OUR LIVES OVER TO THE CARE OF GOD *AS WE UNDERSTOOD* HIM."

The third step then relieved me of obsessive thinking. I learned to *perform* a third step by actively getting down on my knees in the morning and at night to turn my will over to God. I never realized such a simple act could be so helpful. I learned the actual prayer from the AA *Big Book*—the bible of recovery—but just getting on my knees and asking my Higher Power was all it really took to relieve me of so many burdens. I became aware of a Third Voice, that of the Holy Spirit—or just *Spirit*—guiding me through the day. It was wonderful to no longer have to do all the mental work alone.

When I had the spurs taken off my neck in 2003, I had been on a little pain medication in the hospital but was able to come home without any pills for pain. However, I did have a little trouble getting back into the pain meditations I had learned. I could not figure why it was so difficult. So I immediately got on my knees and said, quite simply, "I turn my will and my life over to you, God." I sat back again in the chair and was right away able to meditate. *Voila,* I went quickly into a deeper space. It helps me function during the day with less duress, and it helps me to sleep at night.

I was eventually able to cut my antidepressant and anxiety medication to much lower doses.

THE PLEASURE OF WORKING

To me, living life on life's terms meant doing more than step work. It meant sharing the financial burdens with my husband, so I decided to start back working with something simple, like working in a grocery store. I worked in the deli, salad bar, and floral area of a local grocery store from 2004 until 2005. I learned a lot this year, mostly about human nature.

LESSONS LEARNED WORKING IN A GROCERY STORE

First, and this truly felt like a calling from my Higher Power, I learned tolerance for different racial and ethnic groups—African Americans, Hispanic Americans, Arab Americans, and gays, no matter what their ethnicity. I saw what alcoholism does to lives as I observed alcoholic behavior in a number of coworkers and customers. I was so on fire about recovery that I had to keep my desire to talk to these folks about the miracle of recovery under check. It was just not always appropriate.

I had a hard time understanding some of the African Americans I was working with and serving. Like a lot of people, their mannerisms and speech were just different. One young lady, a coworker, could really boogie and had us all laughing. I was learning from everybody. When I left the store, at night mostly, the parking lot had people waiting in their cars with boom boxes playing rap music. Although I had trouble calling it music, I saw it as an integral part of the African American culture. Black or white, I heard a lot of what I considered bad—or should I call it distasteful?—language. This kind of language no longer shocked me the way it had, but I will never get entirely used to it. It is just not me.

Next—and this is the essence of my feeling I could move on to nursing again—I learned that I was still capable of performing some fairly heavy tasks, even at the ripe old age of fifty-six. Of course, I did not prefer this type of activity, but I could do it as long as I was careful to keep heavy objects close to my center of gravity and my elbows locked to my waist so as not to trigger the weakness in my upper back.

I also picked up a greater capacity to not let people who do not want to cooperate push my buttons, so to speak. I had one incident in particular teach me this. I must avoid, at all costs, letting someone of a different mindset than me drive me out of anger to do a task that will cause me suffering from trying too hard. (Actually, I no longer suffer as much as I get annoyed by my affliction.)

This lesson occurred with a young black fellow named Sully. He was fresh out of the prison scene working with me in the deli. I had asked Sully to please take a ten-gallon can of macaroni salad back to the cooler. The salad continued to sit on the counter. A half hour later, I once again asked him. This time he answered tersely, "No!" Angered by his refusal to cooperate, I picked it up and swung it around to take it to the cooler. By then it was too late and I went through a week of some pretty heavy "feelings." Yes, I was a fragile human being. But I refused to let it stop me. I got through the week of work, reminding myself constantly, *This will not last forever. I can get through it.* And I did.

I have learned the necessary lesson that repetitive arm and upper body work of the heavy nature causes me to become actually confused. It is not a great confusion, but it can be quite disconcerting at times. I recalled nursing in Naples, Florida, during those five years, and I was a poor medication nurse. As a practical nurse I was expected to do a lot of heavy, repetitive work, as well as calculating and administering intricate dosages of medication to patients. This was not a good circumstance for me. I fouled up regularly. Thank God none of my bloopers were too serious, but I had more paperwork to do, filling out incident reports. The only confusing part of deli work was remembering the codes when I weighed different lunch meats.

From February through April of 2005, I learned one more necessary lesson. I learned that I had developed some wonderful boundaries that I did not have before. While attempting to work with one of the department heads—the "floral lady"—at the store, I got the message from her early on that I was to often just, "*Shut up!*" Since I was not used to being spoken to in this manner, I was quite shocked at first. And as time went on, I learned the meaning of a phrase spoken to me by my counselor, Dr. Ramiraz. He said (in reference to staying sober, I think), "Scratch glass, kick ass, and take no prisoners." Well, the floral lady taught me the meaning of *take no prisoners.*

I was walking through her department just to greet her and say good-bye for the day when she took me aside and drew me into a conversation that was absolutely outlandish. I knew this young lady from AA meetings. I stood there for the longest time letting her talk at me about other people's problems in the rooms of recovery. They were women she was sponsoring. When she was done dumping all this information, I walked away, reeling from all the input—input for which I had to ask myself, *Did you want to hear all that, Sylvia?* It is just this kind of third-person question that began to mark my experience at this store. I became aware there was some other voice, some other entity, giving me direction. I'm sure it had always been there, but I had never been so keenly aware of it.

In accord with the third step of Alcoholics Anonymous, I was getting down on my knees morning and night to turn my will over to the Higher Power. For this reason, I was feeling released from the insanity of having to make decisions and work through problems all by myself. The answers seemed to flow through and out of me, often manifested in what I now know as miracles and *A Course in Miracles*. My responses to the seeming babble of everyday life had become, I felt, divinely inspired. Everyday experiences caused a kind of excitement in me because I was close to the Source. Here are two examples.

I worked one day with a woman named Kim who was greatly overweight and known for her foul mouth. She had lung disease and was still smoking like a chimney. I felt almost alone with her in the Carryout Cafe on this particular day because typically she was always *somewhere else* doing *something else* (mostly out back smoking). I was getting very little help from her. The work load was beginning to break me. Naturally, I got very angry with her, even telling her off. This woman always put on a sort of tough girl act, and I found it extremely difficult to talk to her. But then this happened.

I was sitting on break, and the words took form inside me, "*Sylvia, you and Kim probably have a lot more in common than you think.*" This was encouraging for me to hear because I had prayed diligently for her that we might talk and that maybe I might offer her hope. Mostly I just wanted her to heal herself. So, right after my break I returned to our work area, where I found her typically leaning over the counter for support. I leaned right next to her, and I repeated the same words, "Kim, I feel we have a lot more in common than we realize." A conversation between us went on for about ten minutes, and we went on talking after that. Wow, what a miracle!

On that same day, I was on a meal break and heard, *"You need to rise above what you think you feel."* It occurred to me that, according to *A Course in Miracles*, all of what I experience in this life is but an illusion. Therefore, nothing is really right or wrong, good or bad, nor better or worse. Every thought of this life and every "feeling notion" can be dismissed as false. I *can* rise above what I think I feel, for all of life as I know it now is neutral. *"Whew! Do you mean I can stop worrying?"* Ah-hah, yes!

A miracle that I feel is still very slowly unfolding is that the flower lady and I were beginning to talk at twelve-step meetings. There was still somewhat of a boundary there, but I felt both of us realized store business had nothing to do with our individual recoveries—not by far, because recovery and clear thinking come first. Without this, I realized, Spirit would not be able to come through.

Today I am free. I will never go back to my old, sick way of thinking. For this I am so very grateful. In the prayer from the *Big Book* of Alcoholics Anonymous, it says:

> God, I offer myself to Thee, to build with me and to do with me as Thou wilt. Relieve me of the bondage of self that I may better do Thy will. Take away my difficulties, that victory over them may bear witness to those I may help of Thy Power, Thy Love and Thy way of life. May I do Thy will always. Amen.

In 2005, having the ban on my giving out narcotics lifted by the state, I went to work as a medication nurse at a local nursing home. I was not very excited about working in such a place. Nursing homes had always made me so sad—so many helpless, often-demented people in one place. And if they came there able to walk, they were soon put in wheelchairs because of the liability the home felt and the person's inclination to fall. I mean, everybody falls! I was being put through the usual rigors of professional testing and orientation when one morning *A Course in Miracles* and my ability to meditate paid off. I was coming in from the parking lot when I was hit by a wave of worry and fear for what might happen that day. I was being judged, and it felt uncomfortable. So I did a brief, spontaneous meditation, one I cannot take the credit for conjuring up.

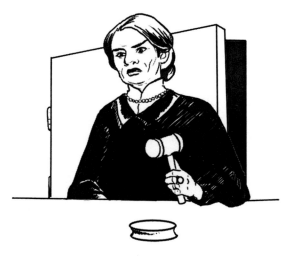

Still standing by my car in the parking lot, eyes closed for a minute, I saw myself dressed in a black judge's robe, coming into a courtroom. Then I heard and saw myself pound the gavel on the desk. I quietly said, "Court is adjourned, and the judge is out." This relieved me so splendidly of feeling judged that I went about the day with more confidence than I had felt so far in this role of nursing. It didn't make me like being there anymore, but at least I could dismiss that feeling. I had learned in recovery that when you judge someone and are pointing at him or her, there are always three fingers pointing back at you. By not judging others severely, I would not be judged. Something else made this job difficult, just as it had in Florida. Yes, it was the old feeling of confusion. At this point I was not fully aware yet of what was causing all the confusion. I had learned from Shinzen Young that pain causes a *sense* of confusion, but it seemed like there was more to it than that. What was it?

I worked at that nursing home only four months. I was so slow and careful passing out pills that they had me monitoring the dining room three meals a day, two sittings per meal—yes, they were twelve-hour days—blah! And the second sitting for each meal was always the people who were less manageable and who often had to be fed. I found myself trying to feed two people at once, and I was still expected to know what was going on in the back of the dining room. One palsied resident even threw his breakfast tray into the wall! I felt extremely liable with so much on me, so I asked to be put in the Alzheimer Unit. It was here where the orienting nurse got me put off the medication cart at this facility permanently.

I *pre-poured* a med; in other words, I had it poured in a medicine cup in the resident's drawer and reached for it for administration. This is a no-no in nursing etiquette, but I was still seeing nurses do it all the time; I just did it in front of the wrong nurse. Realizing I was good with the people, they allowed me to stay on doing activities and patient care for a while. But I got so disgusted with the place that I could not get out of there fast enough. But this still did not discourage me from wanting to work. I soon got work with a home care agency where I did not have to give medications and I could just be myself with people, cheering them, reading to them, and taking them for walks. I enjoyed this because I saw how much healthier it was for these seniors to be in their own homes. The real me shone out for the next five years. I am still at it today.

In 2006 I trained to become something of a new breed in mental health. I became a *peer support*. These are para-professionals who have been and often still are recipients of psychiatric services. They are trained to help others see there is life in spite of having mental illness and to develop WRAPs, or Wellness Recovery Action Plans. This kind of plan helps them to identify when they are in trouble, thus being able to set the plan in motion and identify the help they may need. It is an effective way to avoid becoming emotionally crushed nor in need of psychiatric admissions. Had I such a plan in years past I very well would not have spent so much time in the hospital and away from my family.

In 2007 I went to work for a nonprofit organization in our area called *Keystone Human Services*. These doctors, counselors, social workers, and peer support are the work horses of the community, going into homes and establishments where people suffer from mental illness and helping them become an integral, vital part of society. I soon found myself toting people all over creation in my car, often taking them to appointments or work, all the while encouraging them that they too can have worthwhile, purpose-filled lives. I would have loved to have stayed with this organization, but I was blocked by several problems—mostly my own.

For one thing I began feeling like a taxi cab driver. One of my "consumers," as our service recipients are called, was difficult in that she seemed just downright lazy. I would get to her house at the appointed time and have to go all the way to the third floor to get her out of bed and dressed. I didn't mind that too much. But one time I came and rapped on the door for twenty minutes before her daughter finally opened it for me to come in. Then, the next time I drove up to her house, to my surprise and relief, she was sitting on the porch waiting. I was so happy to see her there, actually expecting me. But when I got to her, she asked me to take her to Wal-Mart to get a new vacuum cleaner belt! That settled that; I was not going to be this woman's gofer.

One woman really put me to the test. It was hard, again, to get her to even open the door. One week I was to pick her up all the way down in Hershey, at her doctor's office. I got to the office only to be informed I had been told the wrong day; I was to come for her the next day. I got there that day only to be told she had canceled. Finally I arranged to see her at her apartment the next day. I got there, and she would not even answer the door. I began to question, like my old friend Angie, nurse, friend, and coworker in Florida used to say, "What am I, who am I—what am I doing here!" But something else bothered me about this job—the departmental meetings.

The meetings were in a rather small conference room with a big table. All the peer supports crowded into this room, including Kathy Ann. She had started with the agency as peer support and now seemed to be running the show. I used to get so angry because she spoke in anachronisms, leaving me in the dark as to what she was talking about. I asked her to speak in a language I could understand, which she would, for a time. Then she would lapse into her foreign tongue again. I saw the valor of her work in what she was doing for the mental health community, but she reminded me so much of my mother; she always had an agenda in front of her. I didn't feel I could approach her as a human being as opposed to a *human doing*.

Something else bothered me about Keystone peer support meetings. Again, it was that little conference room filled with fellow peer support. You have to understand that these wonderful people still had some psychiatric issues going on. Having been in recovery for five years and having pretty much come to terms with my issues—by this I mean I was healed of them—I was annoyed by the behaviors of my cohorts. So many of them had the bipolar thing going on and their emotions seemed to be bouncing off the walls. In addition, many of them were speaking at a fast rate in that foreign language of, again, anachronisms. (Now I am beginning to remind myself of our grandfather, George Allen, when he would pick us up as children at the bus station in Carlisle and reprimand us for talking too fast. *I must surely be the old fogie now!*) But there had to be something else to this situation at Keystone, because I would go into a meeting being okay, and before it was half over, the muscles in my neck and head were so tight that I was in severe pain. What was it in me that made these meetings so intolerable?

Eventually I had to come to terms with my *dis-ease*, as Ms Hay calls it. I had had so much trauma to my upper spine from my years of nursing that the nerves in it were bare and vulnerable. It is, quite literally, like driving a car with all the electrical wires stripped, and this essentially made me like a walking, breathing, living cell phone tower. I picked up their vibes, and they became *stuck; I* became stuck. It was really messing me up. So after only one year, to my dismay, I had to quit again. I was not a quitter, so I prayed, "Please, God, what do you want me to do?" An old Chinese proverb says, "A man can fail many times, but he is not a failure until he does not pick himself up again."

Next I endeavored to do nursing again. And again it did not go well. I was working for an agency that was sending me into nursing homes to give medications and do treatments. The money was just so good, and I was happy I could at least do it. But the consequences, most of which were painful joints and an overwhelmingly tired, older body, got me down— really down. I managed to stick with this for eight months. God knows, I hated those nursing homes. Some of them were the best too. But for me it was truly a nightmare, a fast-moving, impossible trip into *hell on earth*. How could these poor saps let themselves get into such poor shape and such a poor living situation? Again, I could not get out of this job fast enough.

In the meantime, I started to take some pretty strong medication for the pain—yes, the old Oxycontin again. But I have to admit, it actually helped this time. I didn't want it, but it helped. I was glad that at least I did not have to take Klonopin with it, and I realized why it was helping me this time. Now I had the mental skills—the meditations that I had incorporated into my thinking—to work along with the medicine. The only reason I agreed to go on Oxycontin was I knew living with severe pain was, as Shinzen Young taught me, like having a full-time job. And I did not want two jobs.

Having tried my hand twice at nursing since I came into recovery, I decided to give it one more try. In March of 2010, I went to work with an agency that sent nurses into homes. My first and last case with them was in the home of a three-year-old who had what was called "failure to thrive." I loved this little girl and literally threw myself into the case, again doing things that hurt my back. This dear little girl could not eat due to a swallowing dysfunction, so she got tube feedings pumped into her throughout the night and stomach medications injected during the day.

The girl's mother was a spiffy young lady who doubled, when she could, as an EMT and fire response person. When I first began the treks way up to their farm in the boondocks, the mother told me, "Older nurses never work out." I should have thrown in the towel as soon as she told me this, but I'm *not* a quitter, mind you. The dear lady could not seem to remember my name and called me "Whachamacallit" the whole six weeks I was there. Then, to my demise with the agency, after I told her I could not handle the case anymore, she called the agency and told them all kinds of things about me. I am sure she knew what she told them was an exaggeration, but I had been left so alone with the case that there was no one there to vouch for my actual performance. The agency ended up letting me go. I felt horribly defeated by this third and final effort at nursing. I did, however, learn some things about myself.

The mother of my little client told the agency she would talk to me and I would not hear her. Up until this experience, I did not realize how, when I was concentrating, I would not even hear someone talking to me! She also told them I was on my cell phone *all the time*, which was a total exaggeration because I had asked her twice if she minded if I make a quick call. I had gotten some secondary work with the YWCA as a peer support and needed to wrap that work up to give her more of my time. I did not understand the severity of this woman's judgment of me. Looking back, however, it has become clear.

I realized the young mother was in a tight situation. Her husband was working two jobs—maintaining two farms during the day and working as a 911 operator up until two in the morning. I was glad I could help her, but I realize now that I wear my woundedness on my sleeve, often sharing about the miracle of my recovery. I felt it was particularly necessary here because she shared with me that her father was an alcoholic. She was apparently wounded from this. She had a bushel basket of resentments—not just of him but of her mother too. I wanted her to realize, and maybe even pray, that her father might find recovery and someday come to her to make amends, just like I did with my daughter. Well, I must have hit a raw nerve with this dear lady, because here she was slamming me with the agency.

She did, however, make me realize how much my old head injury was affecting me. I was concentrating so intently to keep my ducks in a row. I had to super-think everything so as not to forget what I had just done. That, I have learned, comes from short-term memory loss. I know this now. And I had to find it in my heart to forgive her—it was just where she was in life. I could not go to her because it was against agency policy to make further contact after a case ends. So to mend things in my own heart, I anonymously had a lovely fall bouquet of flowers sent to the farm by a local florist with a note saying, "*Somebody loves you, and believes in you.*" This is *A Course in Miracles* working in my life, and it did help me work through the feelings of rejection and disappointment. The miracle is that today I at least have feelings and can recognize them.

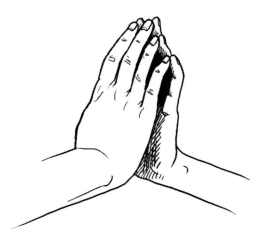

CHAPTER 8

Powerlessness and Unmanageability: *God, Grant Me the Serenity to Accept the Things I Cannot Change . . .*

My journal in recovery is all about the journey inward. You may ask, "Why are you writing the journey inward?" Ever since visiting the chiropractor in August of 2002, it occurs to me no amount of reaching out for answers is going to bring back all the diminished senses I am experiencing from years of traumatizing myself during my work. Constant meditation has freed me of the severe suffering. Shinzen Young, in *Break through Pain*, said, "Don't go to the thoughts for answers." My journey inward is a simple one of acceptance and peace. If there are to be answers to a dilemma, they must come to me.

A common thread in my life was the desire to escape—not just my hometown and the seeming insanity there, as I did by stealing cars with that sociopathic young boyfriend and then riding my bicycle to Naples, Florida, back in the '70s—but also to escape the constant reminder of the near-fatal childhood accident that even *I* could not remember for forty-five years. A fall of nearly nine feet headfirst into a stairwell had left me, unbeknownst to anyone, with bone spurs up and down my upper spine. This resulted in a painful upper back, head, and neck in addition to short-term memory loss. All of this left me thinking, *If I were just to do* something right, *I would feel better*. I was clueless as to just what that *something right* was …

My sense was that something was wrong with my head (which it was, but it was not about psychology as I had thought). This got me into a psychiatrist's office. It was here that I got sicker and sicker with every narcotic he could conjure up on his prescription pad. Prior to that I had used alcohol to numb the pain. It seemed not one nurse or doctor knew how to tell me to live with these illusive feelings. A big part of the agony, like is so often the case with women, was being buried in so much guilt and shame. Then, by God's grace, I learned what I had to *give up* in order to *get back* my life. I gave up all the numbing agents and emerged from that long, dark tunnel. I had truly thought I would not see the light of day again. It was like taking a big, long breath of fresh air after being submerged a very long time under water. I, in essence, became a new person and a testimony to others that even a long-standing, almost mythical condition can be turned around.

In 2002, after flip-flopping through life, trying to dull the pain, and trying six times to end my life, I finally just threw up my arms and spoke into the air, *"Okay, Lord, I am willing to do whatever it takes!"* That is all there was to it—a simple prayer. I came to realize that I was powerless over the substances I was using to numb my body. Instead of me taking the pills, the pills were taking me. And my *life had become unmanageable* because of the frantic, undisciplined mindset I carried around with me all the time. *I came to believe*, as the second step states, *that a power greater than myself could restore me to sanity*. It was a very special realization that I could *turn my will and my life over to God*. Yes, just these few steps of AA were taken in those first few months of recovery. But what happened next, only one month into recovery, was about the eleventh step: *improving our conscious contact with God*.

After only one month of *Break through Pain*—practicing four thirty-five-minute meditations several times a day—I realized it was not God's will at all for me to suffer, and by practicing this diligently, I could be relieved

of the suffering. My thinking had been distorted since childhood, and now relief was just over the next horizon. It was gruesomely slow, but it came.

Growing up in the city and around a business, being hurried along—"Do this ... do that ... get out of the way ... we don't have time for that ..." were mindsets inadvertently planted in my brain. I am sure Mother and Father never meant for this to happen. They loved us. Unfortunately, these things did happen. *Hurry* was the name of the demon that chased me in a childhood game I played up on the farm. It went a little like this: Comically, when I heard a car approaching from a quarter mile down the road, I would dive onto the porch for safety. In my mind, that car was the "devil" and *it* was going to get me!

I know, it sounds crazy, and I would wonder why I played this game. But that was the way my mind worked. I can look back and laugh at it now, but I believe it was this kind of thinking that eventually drove me to such dire straits. I mean, who in their right mind would be awake for three solid weeks? Only someone with post-traumatic stress and/or who had simply never learned to settle herself would do this. That is why I had turned to adrenalin first and then dowsed myself up to my eyeballs in alcohol and later, narcotic prescriptions.

The following was written to share with my friend in recovery, Linda B., and a woman's group brought together by her friend, Nancy Kautz, who stuck with her after being her counselor in the Salvation Army Adult Drug and Alcohol Rehabilitation Center in Harrisburg in 2004:

WHERE MY "THERE" IS:

A reflection upon the essay by T. D. Jakes,
"A Place Called There"

"'I went to the valley, but I didn't stay. My soul got happy and I stayed all day.' Yes, my soul has the power to 'get happy' even when my back aches."
I recall year after year after year lamenting about the severe pain I lived in, not even having a clue why it was there. "God, why must I be so miserable?" I called out over and over. I remember the cloudy and rainy days leaving me

in even more misery. "If only the sun would shine ..." I lamented. I cried and I cried and I cried. The pain drove me into deeper and deeper ... despair until age twenty-one, when I began to pick up the booze.

My history is one of so-called binge drinking. When I was not drinking, I was working up adrenalin at my job to keep me going. The result was many hours of quietly wanting to die or to somehow escape into oblivion. I fantasized gruesomely every night before going to sleep; the fantasy *gave* me sleep!

Being in recovery now from alcohol and narcotic prescriptions for a little over three years, I can look back at a new kind of sustenance. It is an intense awareness of *Spirit*. By means of listening over and over to meditations by Shinzen Young, meditation artist, scientist, and mathematician, I have taken on a whole new way of life. I live my life mindfully and with equanimity. The early-morning meditations I embark upon stay with me all day. I want the whole world to know the wonder of this process—the wonder of no longer living in fear of suffering. Yes, the intensity of my suffering has diminished to almost nothing. I have my life back after over fifty years of losing it. *Praise God.*

Today, my "there" is in my heart as I realize that I can only recognize healing on my own part. But I can lightheartedly look into the hearts and minds of those around me who suffer, be it from physical pain or emotions, offering them glimmers of hope that they too can stop the suffering. All of us were born with a full capacity to get through whatever hardship comes before us, whether it is the loneliness of having lost a spouse or boyfriend or the agonizing pain of having been burned. *We all have what it takes.* However, there is one major requirement.

First and foremost we must keep our thinking clear. Without this, *Spirit* will not be able to get through. We will be lost in the sea of our own thoughts, lamenting over and over, "Why, why, why …?" And although recovery from drugs and alcohol is all about "me," it requires the input of experience, strength, and hope we can only get from a community. The twelve-step programs of Narcotics Anonymous and Alcoholics Anonymous are proven to work, for many thousands of addicts and alcoholics have gone before us to testify to this. This is what has worked foremost in my life of recovery from suffering. Without it I really question if I would be alive to speak of the wonder in my life. Without it I would have, wishfully thinking, thought my way into oblivion.

Yes, as T. D. Jakes cites the bent backs of the slaves in the fields and their spiritual retreats to quiet places, I too find strength in the quiet of morning meditation. I have recognized how driven my life has been. I see people wandering around in a sort of oblivion, almost totally distracted by cell phones, fancy cars, health and beauty issues, and simply not knowing where here is. I see how I have finally found my center, my *Spirit*, my focus. I *see* this, and I want it for all to enjoy. And for today, my "there" is in "*here*."

Thank you for listening.

Wheel: You may wonder how "wheel" relates to learning to meditate and the relief of suffering. One thirty-five-minute meditation in the original four of *Break through Pain* titled "Establishing a Circulation of Awareness" allows the meditator to refocus off the hard fixation of pain and into a moving, living calisthenics of the brain that help him or her to move calmly and serenely **through** the pain **instead of away from** it.

Wheel going around and around, clicking, spinning, driving
me further into life, away from, toward. Where have I
begun, where have I been, where am I going? I just keep
pedaling, around and around … I saw what I saw, I see
what I see, I will see what there is to see. Oh, wheel going
around and around, clicking, spinning, driving me further,
further, further … When I stop, nobody knows; where I
stop I know not either. I just am, I just am, I … just … am.
I … am … I am … I … I … I … am … am … am …

In essence, these words, describing taking a trip on my bicycle, represent what meditation does for the psyche. The turning, clicking wheels and my pedaling, rotating feet break up spiritual blockages. This is why that little girl in a plaid dress came to me happily during walks between the guided meditations. I was learning to walk, talk, and feel like a five-year-old again, before the trauma. I was letting go of all the negativity that had accrued over years and years of suffering. I was finally learning how to live without the misery. And one day early in June of 2002, *I decided to live …*

THE COURAGE TO CHANGE THE THINGS I CAN …

In 2010, after those two more failed attempts at working—one at nursing and one as peer support—I got a really bad chest cold. I knew right away I had it coming. I had no business taking on two jobs, even if they were only part time. I was a glutton for punishment. I had gotten my life totally out of balance in the process. I felt defeated and sickened down to my gut. But right away I turned to *You Can Heal Your Life* and Louise Hay's words for lung trouble or coughing. They were, "I take in life in a balanced manner." In the past, for me, a cough meant weeks of violent hacking. This time it lasted just a week, and the symptoms were mild.

One morning recently, I heard the sound of saws coming from across and down the street. To my horror, I saw men cutting down the nearly 150-year-old buttonwood tree in front of a neighbor's house. Immediately, I recalled my grandmother, still wearing an apron stained from canning peaches, barricading the elm tree on the west lawn of the farm as Grandpa was readying his saw to cut it down. It was the tree her robin was nesting in. I wanted to do the same for my neighbor's tree, but I knew it was not up to me. I still grieve at the loss of this beautiful tree.

I decided that when the neighborhood children and I have our cupcake sale this summer, I will propose the proceeds go toward planting a new tree. I recently heard the saying, "To plant a garden is to believe in the future." Well, surely planting a tree would have similar significance. Ironically, I later found out they cut the wrong tree down by accident! Oh my.

I have attempted a number of *jobs* since coming into recovery, but none of them lasted. I truly believe the old Chinese proverb about a man not failing until he does not get up again. But now I had failed three times at nursing! I had to decide if it was worth it. I had developed such a distaste for it, and for the clinics, offices, and hospitals, all of which I frequented with my own issues in years past. For a while I sank into a kind of sickish lull and even shed a few tears. But then I realized the right door would not open unless I closed all the others. I heard Spirit speak to me, "Sylvia, it is not about having a job; it is all about a *calling*." I knew from having felt happy and fulfilled when I was writing that my calling was to be a writer. The only reason I had not engaged fully in this calling was that I never felt I had anything to write about. Now, at the age of sixty-four, after years of seemingly failed attempts, I am being guided. Now I have a Third Voice—Spirit—speaking to me, and I must stay silent no longer. So here I am, finally, speaking the truth as it is shown to me.

AND THE WISDOM TO KNOW THE DIFFERENCE

Having found the *serenity to accept* and the *courage to change*, now how do I find the *wisdom to know?* Wisdom often comes from the mistakes we have made, but it does not have to be this way. There is a way to move forward confidently and without having had to pay for mistakes ... That way is by plugging into and receiving guidance by that Third Person; yes, nothing less than *Spirit*. Some call this entity God. I don't. I will admit, I am a bit simple minded, but God to me is entirely too big a concept. This is why, I believe, there are so many atheists in the world today. Who can think that big? I can't. But I can think in terms of *Spirit guides* or simply people who have gone before me—and those who will come after me. My mind can grasp this. I recognize, too, that these *spirits* are in a much purer, more rapidly moving energy form. That is why I cannot see them now, but someday I will. We all will.

Thinking back to Miss Francis and *Romper Room* on Saturday-morning television when we were children, she had a magic mirror and could look into it and see all the children out there watching her from "TV land." This fascinated me, and the fascination that someday I will again see the people and animals that were in my life before I incarnated is so exciting and encouraging. Why cut ourselves short? Why live in a tight, restrained life when we can live bigger, all-encompassing lives? Why, why, why? And we would all like boundless energy, cheap gasoline, would we not?

I have found *recovery*, and there has been a *discovery* in my life. That discovery is a whole new source of energy. Having grown up in the midst of a city occupied by noisy, dirty, motor vehicles, I feel another kind of calling. This calling has existed deep within me for many years. I need to at least show the world, and every living being in it, that each of us has an energy source within—a tremendous, untapped reservoir we often let go of in our sedentary lifestyles. The only way to get access to this is to get out there and walk or ride a bicycle. Isn't it a miracle that that seventy-four-year-old man, Ed Mood, inspired me to ride my bicycle to Florida when I was twenty-four? And it is a miracle in the making when more and more of us tap into this resource, our streets becoming quieter and cleaner. We will stop leaving such a big carbon footprint behind us, all the while discovering our bodies are the real *hybrid* vehicles.

It takes courage to strike out and do something different in life, especially if you have never ridden a bicycle. People seem to think that riding a bicycle on a busy city street can be treacherous. This is true. But someone has to start the ball rolling—or better put, the wheels rolling. I wish I could inject some courage into a lot of people to strike out and make a difference in this life, because each of our lives is but one breath in the face of eternity. And an eternity is a very, *very* long time to live. Can we maybe just work on the now? There is a greater cause to find out there. So let's find it, shall we? Let's dig deeply into our souls and find gasoline at zero cents per gallon. We are not powerless over our bodies, and we become stronger with every new effort, wiser with every new experience. Let's live our lives with more *courage to change …*

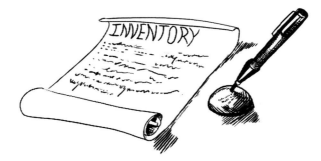

CHAPTER 9

An Inventory

S TEP 4: *"I MADE A SEARCHING AND FEARLESS MORAL INVENTORY OF MYSELF."*

This step took a little more work, and I sat at my computer for long periods, trying to gather my thoughts. To do this step, I had to work through some pretty painful memories of all those years I had suffered in quiet, almost unspeakable pain. There were years and years when I practically threw myself at the medical community with an illusive complaint: "I hurt." I could never put my finger on the source, at least not until my memory finally served me. In doing this step, people came to mind with whom I knew I would need to do some amend-making, but at this point in the steps, it was all about what had happened in my life that created a list a mile long of resentments. As my sponsor pointed out, I had to look at my part in everything too. The fourth step began for me with the following letter to my psychotherapist of twenty-one years.

I did this step practically the first year in recovery, and it was in the form of letters to various caregivers I had over the years. Of course, the primary caregiver was my psychiatrist, Dr. A, and it was basically a chance to let him know how well I was doing.

Tuesday October 8, 2002

Dear Dr. A,

First of all, I want to thank you for seeing me yesterday to discuss my taking the refresher course I have had in mind. Second, I feel the need to reinforce my own thinking. I have become very deliberate in what I do, and this leaves me feeling very, very safe. For example, even our slow bloodhound, Buddy, lately has had to wait for me to catch up when I am walking him. I no longer obsess on the very space I take up. I am comfortable there. 'Tis a wonderfully refreshing way to be.

I feel the need, too, to expound on the effectiveness of my guided meditations, the ultimate "pills" for chronic, severe suffering. I truly suffer very little anymore. Again, 'tis tremendously refreshing! Do you know, I actually catch myself singing, very quietly at much that I do?

Interestingly enough, last evening I attended my first Codependency Anonymous meeting. This, plus my numerous other twelve-step meetings, is supplying me with enough material to deliberate upon for a long time.

I also need to reiterate that when I complete the nurse refresher course, it will not necessarily be my cue to go back to nursing per se. I can only wait until God tells me what to do, if anything, professionally. I do pray to be in a position to help others with chronic pain to find the sort of "window on relief" I have found.

I am very grateful for the time and effort you have spent over the years actively and skillfully listening. I wish, myself, to acquire more of such skills. Thank you for your example. (God knows I bent your ears plenty, didn't I?)

God go with you, my kind physician.

Comfortably yours,
Sylvia Deppen

A later letter to him was not so forgiving. I did harbor some resentment toward him because I felt he kept me in denial by trivializing a dream I had shared with him. If we had explored it a lot sooner, I felt the truth would have come out sooner. He also prescribed all the narcotic tranquilizer and pain medicine. Instead of either adjusting the dose or helping me get off of it when it did not work, he just kept passing me more prescriptions. One time when I was out of Oxycontin way too soon, he passed me another prescription and said, "I shouldn't do this." I asked, "Then why are you doing it?" He replied, "Well, I don't want you to go through withdrawal." It was kind of him but not really that helpful.

I truly wish he had not strung me along like that. He was not qualified to give that kind of medication; he even told me this at one point. So then he gave me to other doctors, who proceeded to do the same thing. Why did it take almost five years for anyone to get wise? It wasn't working!

In the following letter, I gave this doctor a bit of a tongue lashing:

Saturday, April 5, 2003

Dear Dr. A,

I feel I have come to the end of a very long and arduous period in my life. It has been like going through an endlessly dark tunnel—virtually a forty-eight-year tunnel. Now I have emerged, victorious, and by the grace of God can even tell about it. Many would not have lived through such trauma and been able to do this.

Dr. A, you may not recall this, but early in my therapy I related to you a recurring dream. In the dream, I was falling helter-skelter down the stairs. You advised me this was my *"depression speaking."* Now that I am able to look objectively upon the circumstances in my life, I recognize this as my subconscious trying to tell me the real thing—I *had* fallen down a stairway, headlong!

This is not the only dream in which my subconscious spoke out concerning this, but I do not believe I related this to you. I recurrently dreamed of a rabbit—quite the Jungian symbolism—lying at the side of the road with a mangled neck, but its eyes were open and it was still breathing. I realize now that this was the manifestation of how I had felt for very many years but was unable to tell you. I was labeled a borderline personality with a mood disorder, but I wanted to tell you, "I really have a post-traumatic stress disorder!"

The shame of having acted out of order at the tender age of six (I had been warned just moments prior to my slipping unnoticed onto the stairwell ledge), and the resulting pain and embarrassment had to have been such that I knew I had done something catastrophic. This, and having hid it for essentially forty-five years, festered a shame that followed me practically a lifetime. Yes, Dr. A, the shame kept the real reason for my divided and neurotic thinking buried throughout the years I was in therapy with you—I am certain of it now! I feel, too, that over the years I was with you we were so close to this truth, but my lips could simply not spill so much shamefulness and embarrassment.

When I was in rehab at Marworth Treatment Center, I would go to the women's lounge in the late night, unable to sleep, and I would gravitate to a chart on the wall that held the sixth step of the twelve steps of recovery. Over and over I would contemplate, "We were entirely ready to have God remove all these defects of character." Well, Dr. A, this is what I prayed many times over in the coming months. And by my sixth and seventh month of recovery (about September 2002), I heard my counselor reiterate to me, "Sylvia, you no longer have a psychiatric diagnosis!" In my lingering moments of insanity, I practically yelled out to him, "But you can't take that away from me—it's who I am!"

I wore the borderline personality costume a long time, didn't I? But oh how good it feels to have it off. Life is clear and sane; for this I am more grateful than I can express. You were there for me, Dr. A. You saw me through some pretty horrible years. For this, too, I am very grateful.

Dr. A, I have some lingering resentment for having been almost fruitlessly in therapy with you for so long. You have to admit twenty-one years is a long time to be going downhill, as I most certainly was. I have to question whether you ever invested much hope or the benefit of the doubt in me. Do all your clients continue to go down blind alleys, only to find themselves in the end back where they started from? I felt this quite often but failed to speak of it.

It just seems odd that only a few months out of therapy with you and into therapy with a much more interactive counselor, I find myself relieved of insanity. [*A Course in Miracles* made me realize that ninety-nine point nine percent of life is insane, and the remaining point one percent that is sane is the *Spirit* seeping into consciousness.] Do you think it was because my new therapist actually believed in me? It seems this way to me.

You asked me, I believe it was in May or June of last year, "What could I have done differently?" I feel you could have told me more often—either directly or indirectly—that I was, in truth, a whole person and that I had what it took to straighten my life out. You could have reinforced more of the positive characteristics in me. Yes, you could well have conversed with me more. I have to admit there was many a time I felt you were just a warm body in a chair. You actually appeared to doze off at times. I would spin my wheels trying to gain some emotional ground. Do you get what I am saying?

Dr. A, maybe this is an unfair evaluation of you as a therapist, but I am the one who really did the work. And now that I contemplate the circumstances of those years, I feel some resentment. I do not like to feel this.

Dr. Moore, the neurosurgeon, finally removed several large bone spurs from my lower neck and upper back. I know now this caused me horrible distress for a very long time. I worked for twenty-one years as a nurse—actually a manifestation of my codependency—all the while

194

suffering from the chest pain and spasms I could not own. Oh, if only I could have realized this much earlier in my life! Isn't it something how a child will bury his or her shame, all the while trying to live up to someone else's dream for them?

Too often in my therapy I felt I was being spoken to as only part of a person. I believe this was what, essentially, blocked out the truth and kept me a prisoner in my own body and tormented soul. As I mentioned to you too, you might have recognized that I was an addictive personality.

For what it is worth, these are the matters I had to share with you. Thank you.

Sincerely,
Sylvia Deppen

I was a bit ruthless in my criticism of this physician, but it meant a lot of closure for me. My part in it all was that I allowed him to guide me blindly for so many years. I asked few if any questions. And I am the one who let him take God's place. My family, my husband, and just about everyone was telling me to get away from him. But I let it go on—the blind leading the blind. But what I most resented was this man's total dependence on prescriptions to heal me, when what I really needed was just a little positive feedback.

My best counselor, Kathy Russell, who was familiar with the twelve step process, introduced me to Louise Hay and her book *You Can Heal Your Life*. In fact, she inspired me to develop my own affirmation for the often overwhelming spasms in my upper body and face. "I release, relax, and let go. I am safe," became my mantra. I still use it. I also use the words, "warm, soft, smooth, and quiet" and get similar results. But the thought that helped me the most was Shinzen Young telling me, *"You cannot think your way through the pain; you can only feel your way through it."* Escaping it is what had me dwelling outside my body so much, and it did not work. All the adrenalin, the alcohol, and the numerous narcotic prescriptions were false hope, where a change and discipline of the mind was so badly needed.

In the next letter to Dr. A, I took on more responsibility for what happened:

Tuesday August 9, 2005

Dear Dr. A,

Of late I have been rehashing some of where I have been, what happened, and what it is like now [the experience, strength, and hope spoken of in AA]. Part of this is realizing my part in all the years of my illness. Even though I left your care abruptly three years ago, I recognize that you were so solidly there for me for many years. Actually, I brought some pretty fantastic expectations to you, some of which I bring to you here.

I wanted you to tell me how I could think and feel differently and at the same time stay in denial of my original trauma as a child. I could not even look at this; I was continually looking for escape from very real physical pain. The fact that I even had such trauma remained obscure for so long that when I finally remembered it, it did not seem real to me. I looked to you as a father figure, a lover, and yes, even as God. I had lost all concept of God and could no longer even pray. This was one of my first realizations after my head was clear of the narcotic.

Before even coming to you I had been referred to Dr. Jones for hypnosis therapy. This did not appear to be the answer because when I went to him, I could not stop a sudden, surprising flow of tears. From here I was referred to Dr. Barton and then to you. Indeed, I brought you a big package of problems—probably problems I should have been working on for many years prior.

There I sat for the first time in your office in 1980, broken and depleted of energy. To be honest, it seemed like you were the first person who had really listened to me for more than five minutes. Soon, in my mind, the sun rose and set over your head. I was indeed looking for magic. And I realize now this is exactly what you gave me—*magic*. Every time you wrote a prescription for me, you were using a form of it. Unwittingly, I gave all my power to you. My distorted thinking was, *He is going to heal me.* Before getting sober in 2002, I looked for all the most-passive answers in all the wrong places.

Indirectly, you did show me there was another way of thinking that would not cause such suffering. You got me to Dr. Brown for a neurological exam, he got me to Louise Costello for traditional biofeedback, and she finally directed me to Dr. Fink, who was the first person to teach me how to slow my own thought waves through the still rather passive procedure, neuro-feedback. He also gave me my first set of Shinzen Young's *Break through Pain* tapes, which held the keys to a complete recovery.

Dr. A, I think I have mentioned this before, but when I was with you I needed help in getting off all the narcotics, for this is the only way that what Dr. Fink was teaching me was going to have any effect. I remember Dr. W at the Pain Treatment Center telling me he would call me with a place I could go to get off the medicine—but even after I called them back, no one ever got back with me. I was probably ready then but too afraid—or too numb—to pursue it further. It would have been most desirable had you helped me pursue this. You must know, sir, I was on the brink of total self-destruction. It scares me to even think how close I was.

Again, I was in a whole lot of denial and shame-based thinking, and I brought many high expectations to you right from the beginning. For this I am sorry. As I see it now, however, I had to go through all of it—the many hospitalizations, the suffering, and even the suicide attempts—to be the person I am today. My first sponsor in the twelve-step program reiterates over and over, "Everything happens for a reason." Today I am among the "healed healers." Healed healers are healthcare givers who do not put it upon themselves to heal others but rather look to the healing within themselves, and then look to their patients to heal themselves.[x] Yes, my patients today have all the power, not me. Wow, what a weight off my meager shoulders, and what a miracle all this has become for me! Dr. A, thank you for being there for me on the road to becoming the person I am. The struggle made me a stronger person.

Yours truly,
Sylvia Deppen

I suppose one of my biggest resentments could have been that the hospital had made me detox the hard way (i.e., no one even suggested a slow detoxification, as in a modified dose over a long period of time). I had detoxed the hard way twice before but only because I felt the desperate need for help with the pain. I wondered later why no one had ever tried a better dose to help me. However, it is of no use to speculate. It happened the way it happened, and it is probably for the best. As a result of a very, very difficult detox, I was determined to stay off the hard pain medication. And also as a result—I am sure it made me mindful of what taking narcotics could lead to—I stayed off any medication for pain for nearly six years. As a result I began working on those all powerful cognitive skills.

Today, even though I am once again on pain medication, I am still of sober mind. Because I am a quieter, more settled, and grounded person, the pain medication works—like never before. There is a lot to be said for sobriety, if not for any other reason than to learn to think and act soberly. This feels like maturity at its best. I guess it was about time I grew up, don't you think?

My fourth step involved letters to well over a dozen or more practitioners, mostly personal physicians, psychologists, and Dr. A. I had been going to them with my many vague complaints, and then, if I was not satisfied with what they had to offer, I would leave them abruptly. No one was telling me what I wanted to hear. What I wanted to hear was, "I can fix you." But that was simply not going to happen. When I was done with this inventory, I naturally progressed to something a little more heart rending—grief.

THE GRIEF PROCESS

My first year of recovery involved some pretty intense periods of *grieving*. You might ask, what were you grieving? I was grieving all the lost years of feeling any pleasure in life, of missing our little girl grow up, of productive work, and of appreciating having the husband I longed for, for so many years. I grieved, too, that my parents passed away before I could tell them, "It is not your fault." It certainly would have helped had a parent been watching me on that day I went out on the stairwell ledge—yes, indeed. But I was loved and given many opportunities in life because of them. I would have loved to tell them this. And I would have loved for them to see me as I am today. Still, down deep I know that they know. It is because of my recovery that I feel them in my life once again today.

I listened to Stephen and Ondrea Levine's *The Grief Process* on two audiotapes. And another thing that helped was a recording of Tina Malia's *The Shores of Avalon*. In her music, she describes a dream about her mother when she was dying of breast cancer. They were on a boat together sailing to the distant shores of the mystical Isle of Avalon, and as they went, she became the mother and her mother became the child. She then saw her off and into the next life. I grieved and grieved for my mother with this.

I also wrote a letter of appreciation to Pat Taksen, a therapist in the psych ward of the hospital where I rotated in and out so often. Pat had played some beautiful music, a lot of it new age, and I wished at the time that I could feel it. I wanted her to know that finally I could feel music again. What a gift! This is behind the music sessions and meditations I do today as a peer support volunteer on a local psych ward. So you see, where I have been and the atrocities I experienced in this life have made me who I am today, and that's okay.

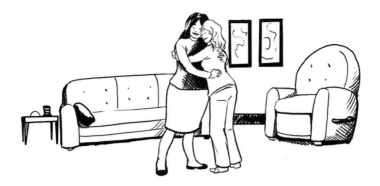

CHAPTER 10

Stepping Forward

S TEP 5: "I ADMITTED TO GOD, TO MYSELF, AND TO ANOTHER HUMAN BEING THE EXACT NATURE OF MY WRONGS."

This evolved over a period of five years. In the first four years, with all the letter writing and attempts to reconnect with the various caregivers that I had left behind in the dust of disgust, I shared the *nature of my wrongs* mostly with that person and God. Then, after making an organized chart of resentments, I finally went to my third sponsor.

Ruth and I sat together in the library of the church where we often met for a women's meeting. I poured my heart out to this wonderful sponsor, crying a bucket in the process. She was a tall, kind of heavy-set woman, and when we stood to depart, she asked me, "Could you use a hug?" The compassion and warmth of her expression drew me into her outstretched arms. All I could think in this moment of extreme release was, *Mother, oh blessed mother!*

Oh, if only my own mother could have shown me such caring and compassion. I knew my mother wanted to but did not know how. This made up for it all. Life felt like it had come full circle. All my resentments and frustrations dissolved into the universe, where all is forgiven. Now my prayer is that someday I get to have someone do a fifth step with me. Maybe I will get to do another myself. But for now, it's enough.

STEP 6: "I WAS ENTIRELY READY TO HAVE GOD REMOVE ALL THESE DEFECTS OF CHARACTER."

This step came about from the moment I first read it on the tapestry of the women's lounge at Marworth Rehabilitation Center. In the quiet of a sleepless night, I had gravitated to it. I remember thinking, *If only God would take this borderline personality and mood disorder diagnosis from me. Was this why my life was so unmanageable, along with the alcohol and drugs?*

In August of that first year was when I first picked up the tapes, "Healing the Unhealed Healer," on *A Course in Miracles*. With this, I was finally able to forgive Mother and to let go of all the wrongs I felt had been done to me: the neglect of not having an emotional connection, the feeling of abandonment due to my parents running a business along with having a family, and the inability to connect with an adult, growing up, in a manner that left me feeling I was an okay person. Only after letting go of these things was I ready for the miracle that was to happen next.

I was with my first counselor in recovery, Dr. Ramirez, when the subject turned to my diagnosis. At this point he looked at me and said with certainty, "Sylvia, you *do not* have a borderline personality—you probably never did."

Phew, miracles really do happen. My sponsor helped me realize later that my behaviors were not so much a defect of character as they were a symptom of the desperation that pain left me feeling. Dr. Ramirez was probably correct; I did not have a borderline personality. Yes, I was a sensitive, rather thin-skinned person with poor boundaries, but the attempts at self-annihilation were really just the call for help that suicide attempts often are. I was really just a person trying to live in the body I had been dealt.

I know, however, that I do have defects. Everybody does. My brother and sister and I talk too much and too fast. I want to improve my listening skills. Now that I have found healing, I would like others to hopefully find healing too. If I listen enough to them, maybe I can help them. I am blessed today with volunteer work because maybe—just maybe—I can show one other person how to heal him or herself too. Really, all

I am doing is giving a kind of extensive, deep prayer, connecting their inner works—the seven chakras, or energy centers in their bodies—to help them feel whole, like meditation does for me. It is all about giving hope—plenty of free, uplifting hope. I don't think anybody can put a price tag on that, do you?

STEP 7: "I HUMBLY ASKED HIM TO REMOVE MY SHORTCOMINGS."

The *humility* and the recognition of *shortcomings* were a little slower coming about than the other steps. I was not sure exactly what was meant by shortcomings. Finally, at a step meeting in my ninth year, it became clear.

I have heard the word humbly mentioned a number of times at meetings over the years. Yes, it takes humility to get down on one's knees and turn their life over to God. I remember how brazen I was when I was drinking and taking pills by the handful instead of as they were prescribed. *A Course in Miracles* taught me, during that first year sober, that for the spirit to come through to guide me, I must first put my ego behind me. Yes, I need to be humble in all that I say and do. I also now know what my biggest shortcoming is. I have for a long time considered myself a *round peg*, and I struggled to get that round peg into a *square hole*. It just never worked. Hmmm … now why do you suppose that is?

Now I have had to humbly consider myself a *square peg*, and in doing so, my life has become much more manageable and doable. A *square peg*, to me, is someone who lacks sound judgment when it comes to practical matters. For my whole life, someone has always had to show me how to go about things. For example, when that neighbor years ago had to suggest mowing the lawn lengthwise instead of widthwise. And in my work as a nurse, I have had to consciously remind myself to take inventory of my supplies: what has to be accomplished, where, and how? If I don't, I am making unnecessary steps and using valuable time. My aging body already reflects such indiscretion, with wearing joints and arthritic feet and ankles.

Yes, pain is humbling too. My pain issues have forced me to take a long, hard look at who I am and where I have been. That is a good thing, wouldn't you agree? Pain tells me I am alive and that is a good thing too, no doubt about it.

STEP 8: "I MADE A LIST OF ALL PERSONS I HAD HARMED AND BECAME WILLING TO MAKE AMENDS TO THEM ALL."

This list was something I worked on very early in recovery. I was doing it in letters to various doctors—there were a lot of them—for whom I had been a complex, problematic patient. Of course, they were well-paid for the headaches I surely gave them. It was my husband and family, however, who came first on this list.

Occasionally in early recovery my husband would remind me of something that happened before recovery, like the fact that the laundry would sit in the machine wet for over a week. Nor did I even try to help with finances. I once gave one of Susan's eight-year-old friends Coca Cola, even though her mother told me she could not drink sweet, caffeinated beverages. The child practically bounced off the walls by the end of our little party. Oh, my! But in time Don saw me improving and taking on responsibilities I use to shirk.

Our daughter was different. She has her own life now and cannot see the difference on a daily basis like Don can, so a number of times I simply went to her and apologized for my old behaviors, to which she would respond, "Oh, Mom, that's water under the bridge. Forget about it." But I could not forget it. Then the day came when I was really able to act upon this necessary amend.

STEP 9: "I MADE DIRECT AMENDS WITH SUCH PEOPLE WHEREVER POSSIBLE, EXCEPT WHEN TO DO SO WOULD INJURE THEM OR OTHERS."

It happened like this.

Since the birth of our little granddaughters, I have tried to spend more time helping Susan around their house. One day she had me help pick up in her bedroom. I had my breath taken away when I walked into the room and saw what looked like three-foot-deep piles of clothes lying around. I had known for a long time she was somewhat disorganized, but this really disturbed me. I have to stay organized because of my short-term memory loss, so it bothered me especially. I cried a little going home that day.

That night Spirit gave me the words I wanted to tell her the next day. Spirit reminded me that when we were on the farm with Grandma and Grandpa, they each only had a few outfits to their name. At the end of the day, Grandma would hang her dress and apron on a hanger in the closet, and Grandpa hung his work pants on a hook. They would never dream of leaving things on the floor. I mentioned this to Susan the next day. I know this was a good thing to tell her. It established what I considered to be old-time, almost-forgotten values. But I wish I had stopped at that and not said what I said next. However, I must first tell you some of the circumstances surrounding their lives.

Our daughter and son-in-law were once involved with a church nearly forty-five miles up the river. They traveled there two or three times a week. Also around this time, they were trying to have their first child. Spirit told me to humbly tell her, "You know, Susan, if you stop leaving home so much and start to do a little *nest building*, you will probably become pregnant." This is exactly what happened too. I don't think I said, "I told you so," but I thought it. I must not take the credit, however, because the prayers of their friends and fellow church members were probably most responsible.

Now, with the incident of the clothing all over her room, I knew at the time she wanted deeply to have another child. But at the time, they were also involved rather precariously with an inner-city Christian ministry, so I told her, "Maybe, if you stopped putting yourself out there so much (e.g., she could play keyboard and sing actively at another church without endangering themselves in the city), you would probably get pregnant again." Well, *Mama*, thou dost say too much!

She lit into me, tearfully blurting out, "Mom, you never taught me how to pick up! You would tell me to pick up my room, and then you never followed through to make sure I did it." She then continued with deep emotion, "Mom, I would die if I could not sing and play for the Lord."

She was right on the money—I had abandoned her those years when she stayed in her room upstairs and I was in my sickbed downstairs. I did a really thorough ninth step this day. I guess it had to happen sometime. We both did some healing. When we parted, we were on good terms. In fact, her last words to me were, "Mom, you don't have to make up for all that. Just be there for me like you have been." This amend allowed me to stop falling on my sword trying to help her—before this I could never get done saying, "Is there anything *else* I can do to help you?" because up until this, I never felt I did enough.

Thank you, God. (By the way, they did stop that ministry and start at the local church. And, she got pregnant! It wasn't odd; *it was God.*)

STEP 10: "I CONTINUED TO TAKE PERSONAL INVENTORY AND WHEN I WAS WRONG, PROMPTLY ADMITTED IT."

This was first explained to me at Marworth, my rehab. I remember joining several other healthcare professionals (addicts and alcoholics, all of us) in the big living-room setting, next to a painted white brick fireplace with a portrait of Dr. Bob above it. Dr. Bob was one of the founders of AA in Akron, Ohio, back in 1935. It seemed so healthy that everyone was talking about their day and people they had to make amends with. The Bible tells us not to let the sun go down on our anger, so I try to stick to this. When Don and I have a disagreement or angry words, I usually go to him and apologize before bed. I sleep better that way; I think we both do.

ANOTHER STEP ...

Of course, the eleventh step has been part of my recovery since early on. I suffer if I do not stay spiritually sound. In fact, today my pain is a gift and a kind of *spiritual barometer* for me. I try to pass this on at meetings when I hear people struggling with painful issues. I also do this by volunteering. I teach breathing technique and working with the seven chakras, energy centers at various points in the body, representing different aspects of a person's life. These centers, when contemplated in meditation, are extremely healing. Before we look at these, however, let's look at how Webster defines "*spirit*," because this term has an interesting variety of meanings.

SPIRIT AS DEFINED BY WEBSTER[XI]

spirit (spir`it) *n.* [[ME<OFr *spirit* < L *spiritus,* breath, courage, vigor, the soul, life, in LL(Ec), spirit < *spirare,* to blow, breathe < IE base *(s)*peis-,* to blow >(prob.) Norw *fica,* to puff, blow, OSlav *piskati,* to pipe, whistle]] **1** a) the life principle, esp. in human beings, originally regarded as inherent in the breath or as infused by a deity b) SOUL

205

(sense 1) **2** the thinking, motivating, feeling part of a person, often as distinguished from the body; mind; intelligence **3** [*also* **S-**] life, will, consciousness, thought, etc., regarded as separate from matter **4** a supernatural being, esp. one thought of as haunting or possessing a person, house, etc., as a ghost, or as inhabiting a certain region, being of a certain good (or evil) character, etc., as an angel, demon, fairy or elf **5** an individual person or personality thought of or as showing or having some specific quality; disposition; mood; temper [the brave *spirits* who pioneered] **6** [*usually pl.*] frame of mind; disposition; mood; temper [in high *spirits*] **7** vivacity, courage, vigor, enthusiasm, etc. [to answer with *spirit*] **8** enthusiasm and loyalty [school *spirit*] **9** real meaning; true intention [to follow the *spirit*] if not the letter of the law **10** a pervading animating principle, essential or characteristic quality, or prevailing tendency or attitude [the *spirit* of the Renaissance] **11** a divine animating influence or inspiration **12** [*usually* pl.] strong alcoholic liquor produced by distillation **13** [Obs.] *a)* any of certain substances or fluids thought of as permeating organs of the body *b) Alchemy* sulfur, sal ammoniac, mercury, or orpiment **14** [*often pl.*] *Chem. a)* any liquid produced by distillation, as from wood, shale, etc. [*spirits* of turpentine] *b)* ALCOHOL (sense 1) **15** *Dyeing* a solution of a tin salt, etc., used as a mordant **16** [*often pl.*] *Pharmacy* an alcoholic solution of a volatile or essential substance [*spirits* of camphor]—**vt. 1** to inspirit, animate, encourage, cheer, etc.: (often with *up*) **2** to carry (*away, off,* etc.) secretly and swiftly, or in some mysterious way **–adj. 1** *a)* of spirits or spiritualism □*b)* believed to be manifested by spirits [*spirit* rapping] **2** operating by the burning of alcohol [a *spirit* lamp] **–*out of spirits*** sad; depressed **–the Spirit** HOLY SPIRIT

Inspire, animate, encourage, and *cheer* are all words that describe why animals are in our lives. Some may consider this a bizarre comparison, but

I have come to believe that even human spirits—*enspiritus animus*—can be represented by pets. *Animus* is the root word for animal. It takes an open mind to accept such a belief. I only ask you try to keep your mind open as I describe having animals before recovery as compared to after recovery. Life just got so much bigger for me; I could not easily dismiss this kind of thinking.

Spirit and My Animals

To look in full at the differences in my life from before and after recovery, I almost have to look at the animals I had during these periods. Growing up in the city, I had a number of grey or brown tabby cats—never a dog, as I so wished—and we had no yard but still managed to raise a couple of ducks and even some rabbits. Up until age six, I totally enjoyed our little piece of Heaven, the roof garden, but after age six, it became more of a prison to me because the back steps were so steep that I did not want to venture down them. I, understandably, developed a fear of stairwells. Our cats, three of them, all named Peewee, always got run over, and I would cry and cry. Mother and Father finally got a golden retriever but not until I was away at nursing school. They did not have him for long though, because he was so nervous he bit a neighbor child. That was the end of that. I had a kitty in Florida but never a dog. That did not happen until I was married, but it was not always a pretty picture early on—not for me anyway.

I needed the steadiness cats brought to my life because nothing in my life felt steady. It was all nervousness and powerlessness over the illusive pain. I had two favorite cats on the farm, Nigga and Shadow, both black, and they had the nicest personalities. But even those cats got run over on that busy country road.

Early in our marriage, the first dog we had was Ranger, a nervous, ill-behaved Dalmatian. As I look back at him, I have to realize that, just as my mother's nervousness years ago fed into their dog's disposition, causing him to bite a child, my nervousness fed into Ranger's as well. I was so desperate for help with the profound sense of suffering in me that I acted out, both with drinking and pill consumption.

We eventually had to have Ranger put down because he kept biting people. The last straw was when he bit me; you do not bite the hand that feeds you! After him came a little yellow lab puppy named Taffy. She especially picked up my nervousness because, by now, I was drinking pretty much around the clock. Proof of how my drinking made things much worse was, at one point, in a drunken rage, I kicked this dear little ten-month-old puppy across the living room. After coming out of the blackout that followed, I lived in deep remorse over this behavior, naturally. Buddy, one of our most faithful and best-behaved dogs, came next. Proof of his dearness to us came one day.

I had been drinking all day when Don came home from work at 5:00. He sat across from me, facing me, and Buddy sat next to him. Both of them were looking at me face-on. We talked together for a few minutes when Don said, "Sylvia, will you look at how Buddy is looking at you?" I looked—he sat staring straight at me, pointing as a dog does, as if to say, "What is wrong with that woman!" Yes, that dog was no dummy; he knew when something was wrong. Of course Buddy was with me on that long, long trip to the rehab in 2002, and he stayed in our lives until September of 2005. We said a heartfelt, loving good-bye to him that year. It was difficult to do, but it was time.

The day before we had Buddy put out of his pain, I got in the car and breathed a little prayer: "God, if you want us to have another dog, I know you will show him to me." Then I drove to the local Humane Society. I walked in the door and was greeted by the daughter-in-law of my best friend. Her name was Niki, and I had forgotten she worked there. I told Niki we were having our little basset-dachshund put down and someone had told me it was best to get another dog right away because this would ease the pain.

I immediately saw the light go on in her pretty young head. She said, "We just got a ten-month-old basset hound in. I will hold him until you can see him in two days." God, evidently, had this one planned for us. When I finally got to see him, the first thing he did was steal the ball cap out of my hands. His name was Bob, and he apparently had plans for us too! Don asked that I let him spend time with Bob alone at the pound before making any definite decision. I respected this and planned to go down at 5:00 to find out the verdict.

All that morning I kept thinking, *He'll never want that dog. He's too big and too rambunctious.* At about noon it occurred to me it was really out of my hands. When I did finally get there, not only was Don signing the papers to adopt Bob, but our daughter and her husband were also there to be part of the process. I was so pleased. I have to say, though, adopting this dog in my newfound sobriety was a little different. Before this I had little concept of what Spirit was in this life. My life now had become so bright and insightful. I had a whole new mindset. Some might call this belief in the Spirit World poppycock, but to me it is real.

When my friend Robert died the night before I found new life, I felt a huge, unexpected absence in my life. It humbled me that he would not make it but I got a whole new lease on life. And as I found out from his girlfriend in Philadelphia, Bobby had wanted to reconnect with me. It was disappointing to us both. But here we were, my husband and I, adopting this basset hound. And he came to us with a name already—*Bob!* I cannot help feeling this crazy, affectionate, *big, bad Bob* the *basset* is some of my friend Robert's spirit revisiting this life, sharing intimate, precious moments with me and Don.

Bobby, as his overprotective mother mostly called him, had never known his father. For all I knew, his father could have been an alcoholic too. And here he was, in spirit and the body of this dog, following my husband around the house and out to his woodshop and back. Don is his master, the man Bob would no doubt lay down his life for. I truly have to wonder, could my husband be the father that my friend Robert never had? Is part of my friend's soul—his spirit—with us in this animal? It's just a thought. I thoroughly believe the spirits of our ancestors and those who have passed before us can visit us in many forms. As I often find myself screaming at Bob, the mischievous, ornery creature that he is, at the same time inside I am thinking, "Welcome back Robert, if it is you in there. I miss you."

In December of 2005, like a little girl again, I wanted a kitten. Don said, "Don't you dare go down to the Humane Society and get another cat!" So I said a little prayer, "God, if you want me to have a kitten, I know you will show him to me."

One day I was coming home from Susan's when I saw a little black creature trying to cross the road! I pulled over and got out of the car, approaching it. It was a little kitten. He ran back into a ravine where he was trapped between Route 283, Lindle Road, and Eisenhower Boulevard, so I went to the Humane Society and got a trap and a can of cat food. The poor little thing had to be starving. Back at the site where I had seen him, I waded through waist-high thistles and thorns, the stickies clinging to my knit, black pants, until I found the perfect spot where he was coming up to warm himself in the sun. If he were to spend another night in that ravine he might have frozen to death. I went into a nearby restaurant and took a seat at the window closest to the ravine.

A young waiter and I talked about our animals, mostly cats, until finally, three hours into the quest, the little guy went into the trap. Then I took him to the veterinarian, who pronounced him to be only eight weeks old. The veterinarian told me the kitten may have a viral abdomen and not survive. I had been learning a practice called Qi Qong, hand and body motions to move and unblock energy, and did some focused exercises with the poor little guy. I called him Survivor at first because of what he had been through. And I put him in a little wire ferret cage by the radiator in our back room, where I knew he would be good and warm. I put a blanket over it and even lit a candle nearby for him. That little guy ate two or three cans of Fancy Feast in one day. When I took him back to the vet, I was told that he really was *twelve* weeks old—three months! He had just been very emaciated.

At first I did not tell Don about our little visitor—I could only guess his reaction. As Survivor got bigger and stronger, because he was feral, I called him Boo Bear. Yes, our new little guy was more like a Halloween cat, frightened of human contact. Boo Bear only comes out now when I go to bed at night, or when the house is empty. He'll come up on my side of the bed and let me give him a belly rub. But as soon as my husband comes in the room or turns over in bed, he darts away. Yes, Boo Bear did survive, and like my other cats, he blesses and comforts me. One such time was while I was working for the nursing home.

I was so slow giving out evening medications that I did not get home until 1:00 in the morning. My neck and head were in full-blown spasms. During the night, I awoke to realize a little black furry thing—Boo Bear—had wrapped his soft, warm body around my aching neck. What a comfort. No one can tell me these little creatures are not here for a reason, because they are.

I am aware of another of our animals having a spirit visiting me. That animal is our young black kitty, Molly. I got her at the Humane Society to keep Boo Bear company in the house. (Yes, I got in the car and went to the Humane Society—tsk, tsk.) Our others were outdoor cats. I cannot help but feel she is the slight presence of my mother back in my life, this time nurturing and taking care of me. I like to call Molly, "The Little Mama," because she likes to lick your fingers. Sometimes she will get up on the back of the La-Z-Boy and comb mine or Don's hair with a gentle paw. She will even try to lick our heads, like she is grooming us. One obvious time of her mothering was right after I had a knee replacement in 2009.

I needed blood work, but the insurance canceled my nursing visits, so I had to go into town to the hospital to have it done. It was a cold, snowy day, and I took a taxi. Getting into town was not bad, but when I wanted to get home, I waited two hours for the taxi. By the time I got home, I was in tears from the pain and exhaustion. It was only four days after the surgery, and I was weak. I lay sobbing on the bed. Next thing I knew, Molly was wrapping her warm, soft body around my right forearm. Slowly I felt the pain leaving me and a wonderful sense of calm coming over me. Yes, it was *Little Mama* taking care of me. I felt a deep sense of gratitude for this unexpected miracle.

Another precious experience happened just two months ago. Don is looking forward to retiring soon, and his demeanor has softened and relaxed even more. We sat at the table facing each other one day when I saw a sadness come over him. I asked what he was thinking. His reply was, "Sylvia, before I met you, I was not sensitive to animals. It saddens me the way we disposed of our old family dog, Trixie, years ago by just dropping her off at the pound. None of us knew what became of her. And I did not used to appreciate cats. Now I find myself worrying that Smokie (our grey outdoor cat) might get too cold outside."

Yes, my husband and I have both mellowed and matured. And we have become so sensitive to one another that we seem to fit each other like soft suede gloves. Not only that, but our spirits seem to have meshed together. We think the same thoughts and laugh as the other says the words he or I was thinking. This is what Spirit is all about: unity and oneness. All are one—one heart, one mind, one body. As we approach the winter of our lives, our egos give way to Spirit; they give way so much that even when we argue, a hearty laugh is not far behind. We struggle—I do—some days because of Bob's mischievous behavior, but never so much as I did with the ill-behaved Dalmatian, Ranger. I have to just laugh off the messes, thievery, and destruction. The only time I did not laugh at Bob was when he got hold of eight ounces of dark chocolate. I worried because he bounced around the house in a caffeine-induced rampage that lasted three days! Yes, life can be crazy, but in that craziness, these days there is always a backdrop of calm knowing that all I or anyone has is the day—yes, just twenty-four hours of *miracle*-filled moments.

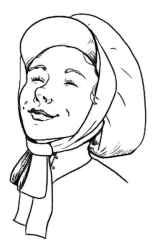

CHAPTER 11

The Diminishment of Suffering and the Eleventh Step

To say that with recovery I no longer had pain would be a fallacy since pain is a part of all mammalian life. But having learned to practice the eleventh step, I was able to reduce the suffering to minimal. In those first two years, 2002 and 2003, most days I meditated six or seven hours. As a result, I no longer suffered profoundly and could function at a near normal capacity, with care not to trigger the places that were vulnerable in my spine. There were, and still are, times when suffering knocks at my back door, reminding me of who I am and what I cannot do—like running, strenuous house cleaning or gardening, and like I did recently, frantically picking up two little girls at once, my grandbaby and her playmate. But for the most part I am free just to be me, whole and emotionally put together.

There are days when meditation is difficult due to excess pain. These are the days when the meditations of prior days click in, helping me get past the hardness of my pain. I have to recognize my emotional reactions to the pain, like writhing and picking my fingers, mostly. Fear still creeps into my awareness, and I remind myself, *This is just for today; tomorrow will be much better, or maybe the next day or the next day … It will not last forever.* As I rest those days in pain, I *breathe* through the area of pain, mindfully putting it together and then taking it apart, and allowing it to move and change. Everything has movement, if only on the molecular level. I allow my diaphragm to work, taking in precious air, and then relax with a slow, deliberate out-breath.

All of life is deliberate—no more mindless, quick movement. This keeps me safe as I remind myself, *There is no time and there are no clocks in Heaven.* Man created those things, and they are only there for us to discriminate where we have been and what we have done, which is nothing, an illusion of a life that only exists, really, in eternity. Tomorrow we all wake up to discover the world is not real; only Spirit, of which we are all a part, is real. If you watch an animal, a cat or a dog, for instance, they don't need clocks, cell phones, or even words; they simply *know* things. When they are injured or in pain, they just trust they will either heal or die, inconsequentially. And *A Course in Miracles* allows me to live in heaven all … the … time … There are no exceptions to this. Each person who comes into my life today is there for a reason, either to help me learn who I am, or to learn who I am not. One thing is for sure: I *am* healed—*totally* healed. If I should smile and you think this inappropriate, then you are the one who does not know.

STEP 11: "WE SOUGHT THROUGH PRAYER AND MEDITATION TO IMPROVE OUR CONSCIOUS CONTACT WITH GOD, PRAYING ONLY FOR KNOWLEDGE OF HIS WILL FOR US AND THE POWER TO CARRY IT OUT."

I had to learn that it is not God's will for me to suffer, that when I keep my thoughts fluid and my chi unblocked, through meditation and mindful, deliberate movement, I won't suffer. Not like I used to I won't! Today, too, I can thank God for the pain, because it reminds me I am alive. And as soon as I douse myself with pain medicine, I lose the opposite side of the coin: **pleasure.** Pain and pleasure are what make life worth living; would you agree? If you are dogged by issues of pain that are unrelenting, are you willing to do the work it takes to realize what a gift it is? It is indeed a source of *purification*, a way to go more deeply into life: a gift of Spirit that we all are experiencing together.

> *Wheel going around and around, clicking, spinning, driving me further into life, away from, toward. Where have I begun, where have I been, where am I going? I just keep pedaling, around and around … I saw what I saw, I see what I see, I will see what there is to see. Oh, wheel going around and around, clicking, spinning, driving me further, further, further … When I stop, nobody knows; where I stop I know not either. I just am, I just am, I … just … am. I … am … I am … I … I … I … am … am … am …*

WHEEL: WHO OF US HAS NOT BEEN DRAWN——REELING, BARRELING——INTO THE TWENTY-FIRST CENTURY? WHO AMONG US HAS FOUND PEACE AND QUIET?

Today, in 2012, this country, America, is in the midst of an energy crisis, but what if the real energy crisis was from within: people driving their fat cat cars all over creation, going places they *think* they have to be, when really the crisis is from within them? I rode 999 miles from Orangeburg, South Carolina, to Naples, Florida, in 1972, but the man who inspired me rode from Pennsylvania to Florida at the ripe old age of seventy-four years old. I am sixty-four years old this year, but I am awestruck I can still get on my bicycle and take the longest hills in one stride, in spite of the years I spent curled up in a little ball, suffering. I believe part of this is because I did it when I was young. Today, are we inspiring the young to use their own, innate, God-given energy to take themselves where they need to go? Have you ever done this?

I have sat at the red light on a main street during rush hour, imagining if all those people—many just one person per car—were on bicycles instead of in a car. Imagine it: people with *quiet, clean* bicycles. There would be no fumes spewing into the atmosphere. The only people in cars would be in fours or fives, or people driving trucks carrying vital commodities, like food, medicine, and large industrial items. That intersection would be filled with people experiencing life at its best, and when they got to where they were going, they would have a feeling of accomplishment, fulfillment, and vitality like never before.

Of course there will be people, too, with handicap placards, declaring handicaps they got from not using their bodies enough—yes, more fat cats with excuses. I have seen people lately pull into handicap spaces at the grocery store and then walk in with not a thing that looks like a handicap. I know not all handicaps are apparent, but I am simply asking that we examine our reasons. Are you one of these people? Is there no way you can kick out and free yourself of this infirmity? There are all kinds of joint replacements available today. And I know often when an ankle or foot is painful, a person can just kick out the arthritic calcium deposits, and go on. This must surely sound callous—does it? But all I am really saying is don't give up too soon! I did, and it almost cost me my life. I am simply challenging the status quo.

Being overweight is a big, big factor too these days. Louise Hay addresses this: "The excess weight is only an outer effect of a deep inner problem. To me, it is always *fear* and a need for protection. When we feel frightened or insecure or 'not good enough,' many of us will put on extra weight for protection."[xii] Here again, is that fear I have been speaking of, that deep sense of inadequacy that needs resolution. If only we could see that each one of us is a walking, living, breathing miracle, that our life work is only to do what expresses love, forgiveness, and acceptance, one for another. The work that makes us happiest is the exact work we need to be doing. Go for it … don't let wages or *shoulds* dictate your life.

We need to move forward bravely. Our ancestors did. They didn't have handicap placards; they were simply brave. Often if we are plugged in and purposeful in life, we forget our afflictions. Yes, there is great peace and serenity to be found in this life when we quit playing the victim: someone looking for the easy road and a soft place to fall. We are quickly becoming a nation of people looking for a *free ride* and cheap gas. It just is not going to happen. Not until we get off our stationary butts and work to get there. When I ride my bicycle, I feel alive. And in spite of terribly arthritic ankles and feet, I get places. Who of us does not want to feel this basic, life-rending kind of accomplishment?

Amen? … Amen.

Here is a message to future inventors of electric cars: go ahead, invent an electric car—it should have been done many years ago, for the sake of our environment and to get us off foreign oil. But real *electricity* and real energy is from within, our bodies and our minds. Can we change our mindset from "take me there" to "I will get there on my own, thank you very much"?

I experience tremendous energy for the simple reason that moving through and breaking up painful feelings in my body have given me a sense of purification. The stuck feelings that used to keep me rolled up in a ball in bed are *unstuck*, releasing all kinds of positive energy that propels me through the day. When I find myself sitting, obsessing in the anguish of *might have beens*, regrets, I need to get out and walk or bicycle to unblock my chi. Today it is like an invisible force propelling me on. And it is good.

Yes, I have, thank God, recovered from many years of suffering, but my body and my mind scream, "Please, please, God, help the people around me to help themselves." I have learned, simply, to pray—my very real and basic purpose in life. What ... is ... yours?

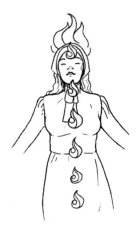

CHAPTER 12

Working with Chakras

I first heard about the seven chakras from a medical intuitive by the name of Carolyn Myss. I listened to her work *Sacred Contracts* and, with Dr. Norman Sheeley, *The Science of Medical Intuition*. Chakras were defined for me as sacred fires or centers of energy at various points in the body. They are attached anatomically to various organs. For me, I see them as indicative of different areas where a person can do some healing in his or her life.

The first chakra is a bright red flame at the base of the spine, and it represents where we come from, a person's birth family and spirits—or *Spirit*—that were there for us before we were born. These spirits loved us immensely and sent us into this life on earth with gifts that are all ours to discover as we explore life on earth. Not only that, they also accompany us into this life, surrounding us with love and guidance whenever and wherever it is needed. I believe we are all spiritual beings having the human experience, and we are all loved, always and forever, because love is all there is. There is no Satan, no evil force, because to even speak of them gives them credence. *I* dare not go there. In Alcoholics Anonymous meetings I have frequently heard, "Religion is for people who are afraid of going to hell; spirituality is for people who have been there." And most of us in the program have been there. We once created our own form of hell on earth.

The second chakra is a bright orange flame and sits just two inches below the umbilicus, or belly button. It represents our ability to support ourselves, our creativity, and most of all, the child in each of us—so spontaneous, ready to live, and full of exuberant life. And inside the belly of each child is a diamond that, early on, is quite rough and dull. With each experience in this life, we polish it so that in our later years, it shines beautifully. This diamond, which I first heard spoken of by John Bradshaw in *Healing the Shame that Binds Us*, allows us to survive sometimes-unspeakable trauma and abuse, keeping us strong and resilient.

The third chakra is a bright yellow flame just above the umbilicus, and it represents our sense of self or self-esteem. It is all about how we see ourselves, and I often challenge people in meditation to see their faces in a mirror in the mind's eye and to *love* that face. The third chakra is about our passion in life too, as we discover what our sacred *gifts* really are. This takes time, and it takes the fourth chakra.

The fourth chakra is in the chest and it is a bright, emerald green flame with a tinge of pink. This energy center is all about our community—the people in our lives. Some people are there for the long haul, but many are there only temporarily. It does not matter which, because they are all there to reflect back to us. When a person is in a room full of people, like in an Alcoholics Anonymous, Narcotics Anonymous, or any such meeting, it is like being in a room full of mirrors. And those mirrors are showing us who we are and what our gifts are. We do not always have to like what the other person says or does—we do not have to like him or her at all—but we do have to love the person, no matter what. Just as everything happens for a reason, every*one* is there for a reason.

The fifth chakra is a bright blue flame in the throat area, and it represents our voice in this life. I know my voice was very quiet, almost silent for years. But in time I learned to speak for myself. A good way to do this is to address the first four chakras—where we come from, our child, and our sense of self and community. We need a strong voice just to survive. We must speak to live life to the fullest. I often, in the years I sang in choirs and at weddings, sang other people's music, and I had an awful time expressing it in the proper time, words, and notes. Then one day I woke up and realized the music was just in my words, and this was enough. In this way, each one of us has a *song* to sing, and I need to hear yours (isurvivedchronicpain@gmail.com).

Shinzen's *Expanding and Contracting with the Breath* is about the fifth chakra. This meditation especially helped me heal of being claustrophobic. I had nightmares of being trapped in a small room. After practicing this for a while, I realized that if someone were to trap me in a small box or coffin, I would not panic. Instead, I would go into this deep, slow breathing … And by doing so, I could survive for a long time in that box. And if I did not survive, I would at least not suffer being snuffed out. Again, death is the ultimate lie. I have to watch myself at funerals that I don't smile too much. But I do chuckle to myself because one truly need not mourn.

The sixth chakra is a bright purple flame in the head, where I have heard reference to a *third eye*. Here is the strategic command center, where we align the other five chakras and get prepared for the seventh. I like to remind people that if there is a need for a question in their lives to be answered or if there is a need for direction, this is where you can *put it out there*, present it to Spirit. And even more important than asking, we must expect an answer. Answers and direction most frequently come before we are even aware of a question. A deeply rooted, intuitive person is open to these answers. That is why I suggest practicing meditation on a regular basis, because, "*A day without meditation is like carrying an unopened gift all day.*" So why not open yours?

A flaming white crown, the seventh chakra, is what connects us to the heavenly realm, Spirit. Finally, when all the chakras are aligned, we can begin the healing process, and part of that process is to pray for the people around us and in our lives, because all are One. When one of us is suffering, others feel this and can suffer too. But remember, life as we know it on earth is but one breath in the face of eternity. One person is but a speck in God's eye, an inseparable part of Him. And from this standpoint, what a view!

One of Shinzen Young's four meditations in *Break through Pain* is called, "*Working with Space.*" This marvelous meditation was so healing for me that I do it regularly now. I can do it while driving a car—with my eyes open, of course—or while in an interview for a job or any stressful situation, like heavy traffic or when I am amongst people who are acting out difficult emotions. There is no place I cannot do it. *Voila*: a comfortable place inside that no one can take from me! *Working with Space* gave me a tremendous sense of inner freedom. It has opened me up for learning too.

This place of comfort that opened up inside me early on was the reason I found so much sanctity in one of the AA meetings, my Fortieth Street Wednesday night women's meeting. This was a group of seven or eight women, many of them in early recovery and a few with some good time under their bonnets, who first introduced me to the twelve steps. I recall one woman older than me by more than a decade. Her name was Rachael, and she was nearly seventy years old when she found sobriety. Rachael, a tall, black woman, spoke of God having "removed the *taste* of alcohol" (i.e., she no longer had the desire to drink). I heard this said by others too.

It was the same for me. I did not even want the pills anymore. Now, over nine years later, I am still of sober mind. Nearly three years ago, because my spine suddenly shifted from some surgery, I was forced to go back on Oxycontin. I stalled for months, not wanting to go there again. But in the end, not desiring to play the superhero, it was a question of being able to work or not. Living with severe pain alone is a full-time job, so I conceded. But I was surprised and gladdened to realize the Oxycontin actually worked for a change. I finally got a doctor to work with me on it, adjusting it to a viable dose. For this reason, I can work. But it is imperative that I maintain regular periods of relaxation and meditation. It does not take long periods, as it did those first two years. A state of meditation comes easily now.

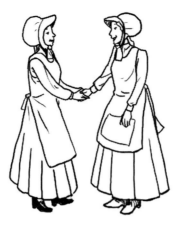

CHAPTER 13

And the Last Shall Be First

STEP 12: *"HAVING HAD A SPIRITUAL AWAKENING AS THE RESULT OF THESE STEPS, WE TRIED TO CARRY THIS MESSAGE TO ALCOHOLICS AND TO PRACTICE THESE PRINCIPLES IN ALL OUR AFFAIRS."*

This step began only a few weeks after I returned home from rehab. I connected right away with another, younger woman, Niki, in the outpatient drug and alcohol program I was in. We kept each other sober. I would run all the way to Mechanicsburg, twelve miles away, to pick her up, and then take her home after the IOP or the meetings we attended together. I put a lot of miles on my little red Cavalier that year.

I was by nature gregarious, so this came easily to me. What did not come easily was that she was recovering from street drugs and I wasn't, and she had a lot harder time staying sober. There is a difference in recoveries— recovery from prescriptions, where the substance of choice for numbing is not readily available, I believe to be easier. On the other hand, street drugs are available by just going to the curb and soliciting. The last I saw or heard of Niki two years later, she was still struggling. It is hard, too, because I could not identify the stressors in her that kept her picking up a drug. I wanted to scream at her, "Niki, just settle yourself!" But how much good would that have done? She was younger than me by over twenty years, single, and scrounging to get her life together. On the other hand, I had been married almost twenty-five years and my life was centered around a husband and family.

It is so easy to judge a person, but I feel if you have not walked a lifetime in that person's shoes, there is no room for judgment. I have observed many a young person in recovery over the years floundering like Niki. When I do, I cry out inside, "Please, please, just learn to meditate—get quiet and comfortable inside." Again, we all have this place of genuine comfort available to us, and that *Third Voice* is waiting for us to merely connect and become part of a bigger place. I call this Spirit Place: an invariable, constant state of being in *Heaven*. *A Course in Miracles* tells us everyone is always in a state of grace. Call it what you like, you are there.

I have heard it said by many a twelve-stepper, someone who relishes recovery meetings, "I walked into this meeting feeling rather discouraged and miserable, and I walked out feeling I was floating two feet above the floor." I cannot hear the *Promises* enough from "Into Action" on page 83 of the *Big Book of Alcoholics Anonymous*:

THE PROMISES

If we are painstaking about this phase of our development, we will be amazed before we are half way through. We are going to know a new freedom and a new happiness. We will not regret the past nor wish to shut the door on it. We will comprehend the word *serenity* and we will know *peace*. No matter how far down the scale we have gone, we will see how our experience can benefit others. That feeling of uselessness and self-pity will disappear. We will lose interest in selfish things and gain interest in our fellows. Self-seeking will slip away. Our whole attitude and outlook upon life will change. Fear of people and of economic insecurity will leave us. We will intuitively know

how to handle situations which use to baffle us. We will
suddenly realize that God is doing for us what we could
not do for ourselves.

*Are these extravagant promises? We think not. They are being
fulfilled among us—sometimes quickly, sometimes slowly. They
will always materialize if we work for them.*

ON SPONSORSHIP

Sponsorship is twelfth-step work, and sometimes a real challenge. It is a
challenge because so many people either just don't want sobriety or they
don't grasp a hold well enough. I have worked with a number of people in
recovery over the years, most of whom just either disappeared for good or
came back to recovery after a period of relapse or multiple relapses. It is
hard to watch.

One young lady, Ellen, age twenty-four and about my age when I took
off for Florida with my sociopathic boyfriend, was my sponsee for a period
of six months. I followed her from a recovery house in Harrisburg, to
Dauphin County Prison, to a rehab, followed by a stay on a psychiatric ward
in Danville, Pennsylvania, and ending in another recovery house in Carlisle,
Pennsylvania. Finally, I hoped to get to work more with her, but something
changed in me—something I was unaware of.

I went from being a firm but supportive sponsor to being more of a
frightened mother, worried for her child. She picked it up right away, and I
was soon added to her resentments list. I cannot help feeling she thrived on
this list. All alcoholics and drug addicts tend to keep such a list. Of course
I had no intention of becoming a resentment of hers; it just happened. I
realize now that fear replaced love entirely; they cannot coexist. That was
why it went bad. She eventually picked a drug up again and it literally tore
my heart out.

My sponsor said not to blame myself, but I do to some extent. I must
take credit where credit is due, or as in this case, *discredit* where discredit
is due. Had I worked one-on-one with her and stayed in the upper four
chakras—where there is simply love, speaking truth, actively listening, and
sharing inspiration—I could no doubt have really helped her. Instead I was
shrouded with fear of where she was coming from, which was a sick mother

and father, the vulnerable child I saw in her, and a lack of passion for life. I have to learn from this experience, and hopefully Ellen does too. I pray someday to see her again, and the amends will no doubt be two ways.

This experience tells me to be a *healed healer*.

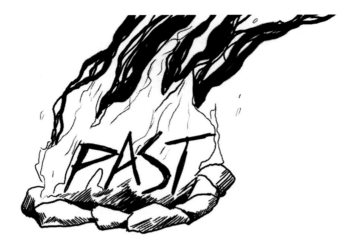

CHAPTER 14

A *Healed* Healer

A sponsor needs to be a *healed* healer and shine a light on truth. The ego's plan of forgiveness entails shining a light on the nightmare to show what a *miserable sinner* both the sponsor and sponsee are. This just never works. What really works is to show that none of what happened in the past is real—absolutely none of it! When you think about it, nothing lasts. It is all past tense and gone. What really matters is that we listen for our inner voice, the voice of the Holy Spirit. *The Course* puts it this way:

> When God said, "Let there be light," there was light. Can you find light by analyzing darkness as the psychotherapist does, or like the theologian, by acknowledging darkness in yourself and looking for the distant light to remove it, while emphasizing the distance?[xiii]

A sponsor needs to have a clear mind, which comes from true sobriety. When that mind is clogged with its own issues, a negative self-image, or feelings of inadequacy and doubt, that person cannot be a good sponsor.

True, even the mind of someone who has been sober for ten or twenty years can be clouded this way. But if that person spends enough time clearing his or her mind through meditation—time spent in quiet contemplation and prayer—he or she will be a good sponsor. There needs to be clarity of *knowing* as opposed to simply *perceiving*. Knowing comes of the journey inward, and perception, the bare realization of facts, comes of constantly reaching outward, the journey outward.

Many of us have trouble handling quiet time. I know I often do. I catch myself always wanting the television on when I am at home alone. And just like the young man in the movie *Home Alone*, this begets mischief. It is only when we are able to click the off button on the remote and go into extended, deep quiet that we shine a light on truth. The truth is that not one of us is ever but a breath away from our Creator. Not one of us lacks this internal navigation system. Just like the young man in the movie *Flight of the Navigator* in the nineties, we are at the helm of our own space craft and able to guide it safely to its destination. But just what is that destination? Where are we headed?

We are *all* headed back to where we came from, on the other side of that *veil of forgetfulness* that the Course talks about. I have noticed, when at the end of an AA meeting the person closing it says, "Let us have a moment of silence for those sick and suffering alcoholics (or drug addicts) still out there, followed by the Lord's prayer." that *moment* only lasts twenty seconds, if we are lucky. What happened to the other forty seconds? Again, why are we so reluctant to hesitate? Are we afraid of what will happen to us with a long pause? Are we afraid of what we will find out? The key word here, again, is afraid or fearful. And because we are in fear, we are canceling out the love we need to leave the meeting with the faith that all will return safely (i.e., no more relapse). Heaven knows we do not need relapses!

The Course also says, "By their fruits ye shall know them, and they shall know themselves."[xiv] Just as it speaks of a *true therapist* being someone who lets healing be, a true sponsor is someone that lets his or her sponsee heal themselves. No one can really heal another person. Again, it must happen from the inside out. I have found a really good way to end a meeting is to allow for that full minute of contemplation and *meditation/prayer*. In that moment, I like to get a visual (i.e., a picture in my mind) of one very large hand holding the whole room full of recovering people up, up, up ... into a higher realm, where they are all safe. We are all safe, I know today, **and** no matter what we will be okay.

This may sound like a ridiculous blanket statement, but it is true. We **are** all safe. Even if one of the group goes out and picks up alcohol or drugs, and dies as a result, they will be okay. Because just as death is the ultimate lie, love is the only entity that gives back many, many times over—that love is what makes us safe.

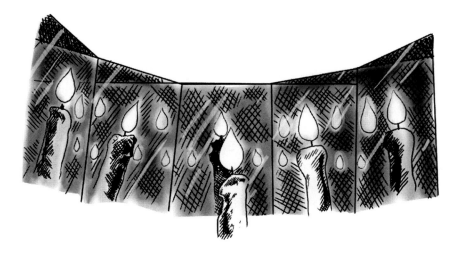

CHAPTER 15

Meetings: A Room Full of Mirrors

"*BECAUSE I WILL TO KNOW MYSELF, I SEE YOU AS GOD'S SON AND MY BROTHER.*"[xv]

The first twenty-four years of our marriage were, on my part, a constant desire to self-annihilate and an uphill battle to overcome a deep sense of ongoing pain that kept me in the suffering mode. It tested everybody's patience. My parents died years before the realization of the nature of my affliction surfaced. I was never able to enlighten them about my fall as a child, which would have helped explain the bizarre behaviors I had exhibited. None of it was their fault! My husband just stood by me in spite of it all. Our daughter had to have been glad to marry and get out of the house. I so wished I had had more a part in her later years growing up and her preparation for married life. But we all survived by God's grace.

My dream ... *click, click, click, click* ... revealing what had happened to me ... *click, click, click, click* ... finally led me to do what I needed to do to heal. The truth ... *click, click, click, click* ... finally did *set me free* ... Today

I have found a steadiness and balance not just in riding a bicycle but in my thinking and behavior too. I also have had to surrender to the fact that I am not only severely upper spine damaged, thus rendering me vulnerable to injury, but I am head injured too. No one wants to have to face this kind of personal injury. But in facing it I am finally able to accept it fully. Don't we all need this kind of clarity?

Besides Shinzen Young's *Break through Pain*, I was inspired by various other artists. Another was Stephen Levine in *Merciful Awareness*. He and his wife Ondrea are hospice workers. I enjoyed the meditations in Wayne Dyer's *It Is Never Crowded along the Extra Mile*. Real relief from suffering is not a complicated matter at all. Simple rotating, moving thoughts are the most effective relief anyone could need. Many times in recovery I have heard reference to "KISS"—keep it simple stupid. I recall myself intellectualizing, while at the same time wondering why I was so miserable. The best things in life really are the simple things: love, smiling at the person in front of me and reaching out and inquiring of them from the heart. Instead of escaping our challenges, shall we dive headlong into them? Are we ready to throw up our arms and say, "Whatever it takes, Lord"? Because when this happens we open ourselves to the real miracles waiting to take place. Meditation, not medication, is an excellent way to release your dream, to unwrap the gift of Spirit in your day, your life, and that of those around you.

If you have suffered a very long time there may be a lot of anxiety and depression built up inside. If this is the case, as it was for me, psychotropic medicine may be in order. But once a steady improvement or plateau is reached, even this can possibly be reduced or stopped—but only after finding steady improvement and under the watchful eye of a therapist. Above all I encourage you to practice these meditations diligently. Are you gifted with enough desperation to really stick with this process? Because if you do, you will release bounty in your life directly equivalent to what you put into it. We can all be healed in ways we never imagined. So, just do it. *Just do it.* And while you are at it, ride a bicycle, or just walk.

> We are so busy; we don't want to do so many things. We want to know just one thing that we can do to get closer to the happiness we seek every day. I think that moving around with mindfulness, walking mindfully, may be what

we propose as a gift, because we move a lot during our daily life. If you want to go from here to there, even if you need only to make five or six steps, and if you know how to make these steps mindfully, that can already be very helpful. You walk to the garage, enjoy every step you make. Don't think of anything else, just enjoy walking. You walk to the office, to your workplace or to the dining hall: Every step you make should bring you back to the here and now so that you can enjoy what is going on. I think *if all people on Earth were to know how to enjoy walking mindfully, that would transform the Earth and society already; because everyone would have the secrets of becoming more mindful, everyone would know how to enjoy each step they make.*

—Thich Nhat Hanh, Vietnamese Monk[xvi]

I thank all my readers for *listening*. May you have heard what you need to *know*, because you deserve clarity of mind, soundness of body, a loving community around you, and an all-around *spirited* life. This is the way we were intended to be.

I am including an appendix at the end of this book with a suggested format for twelve-step meetings of Chronic Pain Anonymous. The steps have been slightly rewritten but only enough to change the focus from drugs and alcohol to chronic pain and illness. No one chooses to be powerless over these things, but when it happens it is good to at least know that release from suffering can be found. Anonymity is highly suggested due to the personal nature of such a meeting.

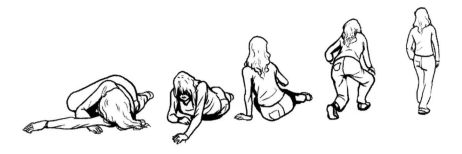

As I Look Back

"*Come unto Me, My children, once again, without such twisted thoughts upon your hearts. You still are holy with the Holiness which fathered you in perfect sinlessness, and still surrounds you with the Arms of peace. Dream now of healing. Then arise and lay all dreaming of peace down forever. You are he your Father loves, who never left his home, nor wandered in the savage world with feet that bleed, and with a heavy heart made hard against the love that is the truth in you. Give all your dreams to Christ and let Him be your Guide to healing, leading you in prayer beyond the sorry reaches of the world.*"[xvii]

As I look back, it has been a hard, mindless struggle with not just chronic pain but a subtle head injury that increased my physical workload many times over the years. The more I *resisted* what I felt, obsessing all the while in my mind, the less able I was to cope. Indeed, living this way can be exhausting. If in reading *Wheel* a person gets no other message, I would want them to know the following:

If chronic pain or illness has you down, don't give up too soon; I did, and it almost cost me my life. Don't wait until you have lost your life by lying and sitting around in dreaded remorse when you can engage that precious mind in constructive, affirmative thinking—yes, mind*ful*ness instead of mind*less*ness. You are indeed the master of your own destiny, the captain of your ship. Bring that ship back peacefully into harbor, and note the treasures you have already gathered into the hold. Yes, thoughts can be turned into gold, so start spinning today: *You can do it!*

232

I have found too that handwork, like sewing for me, keeps me engaged and happy. What can you do with your hands? I believe the saying is, "*Happy hands, happy heart.*"

I am a licensed practical nurse, and I made great strides to better my skills in this regard, only to be discouraged over and over due to the distractibility encountered with pain and the short-term memory loss. For this I feel more like the letters LPN stand for *let's play nurse*—as if I never put that plastic, play doctor's kit away and was still a child playing with the idea. I still crave reading, but this late in life I have felt discouraged by the little I have read and the number of volumes still on the bookshelf of my mind. With this I remind myself that there will be other lives. And in these lives, Lord willing, you will get to read any and all there is to read, Sylvia. Yes, *life goes on* … and with that perspective, I have all the time in the world. Besides, knowledge is absolute, so why obsess about it?

I have also learned the power of gracious thoughts, that when I live in gratitude for the little things—and the big—I live a much richer and more abundant life. I am indeed grateful that our daughter's marriage, in spite of my negativity and lack of feelings throughout the event, has turned into a good life for her. Of course, bad things still happen on occasion, mostly just people pointing fingers and quickly judging. Who would not be affected by this? But today I see this kind of often-blatant attack as simply a *call for love* in a world full of nasty ego. And my thoughts are about this: bring 'em on, I can take it. But don't expect me to fight back, because today my life is about forgiveness, not attack. And oh, the peace of mind this affords me. Try it—you'll like it!

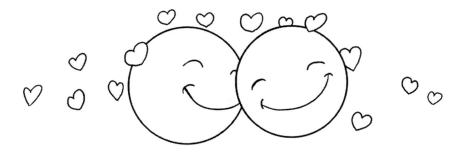

Yes, smile in the face of adversity,
and the world will be yours.

Finally, where once I had no brakes, I learned
to tell myself, "Now is a quiet time to let peace
become me. It is okay to be still, because ...
'*Nothing real can be threatened.*
Nothing unreal exists.
Herein lies the peace of God.' "[xviii]

The author, once again, was able to get off the Oxycontin, this time through a slow detoxification. She did so not to prove she was a super-hero, but rather as a confirmation that the best comfort is natural comfort. Peace, she knows, is a frame of mind, not a mind in a frame; e.g., dependent on outside circumstances. All it took for her was a more constant state of meditation; for love is the elixir that heals all life. So be it.

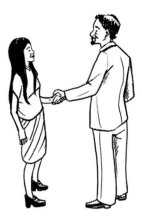

Appendix

CHRONIC PAIN ANONYMOUS[XIX]

Hello, my name is _____ and I have suffered from chronic pain and illness.

Chronic Pain Anonymous is a fellowship of men and women who share their experience, strength, and hope with each other so that they may solve their common problem and help others to recover from the disabling effects of chronic pain and illness. We believe that changing attitudes can aid recovery.

The only requirement for membership is a desire to recover from the emotional and spiritual debilitation of chronic pain or illness. There are no dues or fees for CPA membership. We are self-supporting through our own contributions. CPA is not allied with any sect, denomination, politics, organization, or institution; it does not wish to engage in any controversy and neither endorses nor opposes any causes.

Our primary purpose is to live our lives to the fullest by minimizing the effects of chronic pain and illness in our lives and helping others to do the same. We do this by practicing the Twelve Steps, and welcoming and giving comfort and understanding to each other.

Half measures avail us nothing.

Here are the steps we can take:

1. We admit we have been powerless over the pain and illness—that our lives had become unmanageable.[1]
2. Came believe that a Power greater than ourselves could restore us to sanity.[2]
3. Made a decision to turn our will and our lives over to the care of God *as we understood Him*.[3]
4. Made a searching and fearless moral inventory of ourselves.[4]
5. Admitted to God, to ourselves, and to another human being the exact nature of our wrongs.[5]
6. Were entirely ready to have God remove all our defects of character.[6]
7. Humbly asked Him to remove our shortcomings.[7]
8. Made a list of all persons we had harmed and became willing to make amends to them all.[8]
9. Made direct amends to such people wherever possible, except when to do so would injure them or others.[9]
10. Continued to take personal inventory and when we were wrong, promptly admitted it.[10]

---

1 "God, grant me the serenity to accept the things I cannot change, the courage to change the things I can, and the wisdom to know the difference."

2 Are there miracles and a sense of magic in my life?

3 But what will carry us when we do?

4 What it was like in our suffering, what happened, and what it is like now?

5 Am I learning to trust myself, and can I learn to trust another person, conscientiously addressing any and *all* denial?

6 I am finding and identifying my defects, and I sense when they are finally gone.

7 Am I addressing possibly dysfunctional behavior? The proof is in the pudding.

8 This *is* where I begin to find the courage to change the things I can.

9 God give me the wisdom to know the difference; but can I first forgive myself?

10 There is significance, at times, in standing back from or outside of a given situation.

11. Sought through prayer and meditation to improve our conscious contact with God *as we understood Him*, praying only for knowledge of His will for us and the power to carry it out.[11]

12. Having had a spiritual awakening as the result of these steps, we tried to carry this message to others with chronic pain and illness, and to practice these principles in all our affairs.[12]

Ten minutes of music [optional] *and silent meditation or a meditational reading, followed by respectful sharing.* Feel free to share, without interruption, sit only thinking for a few minutes, and/or pass to someone else.

In Closing

Having invested this little bit of time in listening and sharing with others, shall we take these thoughts with us and keep each other in prayer throughout the coming week? Shall we take time at regular intervals throughout each day to pray for not only our own *happiness, health,* and *wholeness,* but that of each member here? Shall we pray for the *holy instant* of release for us all? For we all are One—one with each other, one with the Father, and one with Spirit, always and forever. *Amen.*

***Remember, who you see here and what
you hear here stays here.***

---

11   Step 3, Step 3, Step 3…This is, morning and night, getting down on my knees, if at all possible, and turning my will over to Him. Only this will show how truly functional meditation and prayer can change my life.

12   Am I daring to dream for myself? Am I encouraging others who need it in order to help them change their lives—sometimes quickly, sometimes slowly?